Improving Healthcare in Canada

George O. Obikoya

Table of Content

Executive Summary	3
Introduction	6
Of Rights and Health	8
On the Mimicry of a Lamb	37
The Wait Times Issue	66
A Political Philosophy of Health	95
The Future of Private Health Insurance	126
On An Appeal to Nature	155
A New-Stone Age	180
Conclusions	204

Executive Summary

Healthcare delivery is about to undergo its most dramatic transition in recent times, the undercurrents of whose arguably staccato history, are legion. Not only is health spending increasing substantially in many countries, it is apparent that not even developed countries could sustain indefinitely an ever increasing health budget. This is of major concern to all healthcare stakeholders not least with the benefits derivable from the increased health spending often uninspiring given the several questionable key health indicators in many of these health jurisdictions.

That health systems worldwide would therefore need to seek ways to provide qualitative health services simultaneously curtailing spiraling healthcare costs is not in question. Indeed, are health systems, not better off actually able to reduce health spending in the process? Considering the realities of our times, the tendency for seemingly disparate domains to interface in the healthcare delivery enterprise would increasingly spawn sophisticated value propositions with the potential to impel the achievement of these objectives.

The onus is on health policy makers, in collaboration with healthcare consumers and other healthcare stakeholders to establish the mechanisms to activate the motion whose impetus would constitute the catalyst that virtually all health systems need to meet the requirements to survive, let alone thrive in a milieu of more acute healthcare consumer awareness of acceptable standards of care. Yet, the potential implications of relentless budgetary pressures on the nature and quality of service provision in many health jurisdictions call into question their ability to meet these requirements.

The search then, subject to the acknowledgement of the imperative for change would be for its accelerators, which is what this e-book endeavors to do, and in attempting to accomplish which it delves deep into the fundamental undercurrents upon which the inevitability of the motion of health systems, including its pace and direction, depends. The e-book explores the curious bimodality of inevitability and change inherent in this motion, in all its facets, which inquiry posits the imperative of health systems operatives and indeed, all health stakeholders to appreciate fully the interplay of the symbiotic dyadic driving healthcare delivery through its transitions.

Even more significantly, it situates this interplay contextually within the larger framework of the evolution of society and its economy, and its ramifications within and without this context. This is in keeping with a vigorous re-conceptualization of the elements of the transactions that run through every dimension of both as they operate in tandem to propel the grand motion of which healthcare delivery is a part, in which direction the accretion of forces essentially dictates. Furthermore, as is evident in our applications of this heuristic to the Canadian health system, it is this very propensity for channeling the healthcare delivery process that underscores the need for even further exploration crucial to the potential for ongoing quality improvement implicit in the exercise. It is also clear from our examination that the activation and pursuit, or otherwise of this potential, is just as important, as it in turn determines in the main, the path of the transition that the country's health systems eventually tread.

Introduction

Canada's Medicare represents both aspiration and imperative in equal measure. The question of the recognition of the former attribute is essentially settled, that of the latter though, moot. It is clear that Medicare has to evolve in the appropriate direction as indeed, any other program in the country has, not just to deliver on its promise but also to maintain its relevance to its stated objectives. This evolution, its nature, and characteristics, and the factors that promote or hinder it, are some of the issues, among many others that we would address in this e-book, and relate to the place of the country's health systems in the overall scheme of its existence and indeed, of its progress.

We would first revisit the underlying concepts of the value-base of contemporary approaches to healthcare delivery, and in relation to the country's present approaches, explore the potential for reformulating the value propositions therein embedded and in general, in contemporary healthcare delivery approaches relative to the demands of our times, and those anticipated in the future. The goal of this exercise being to elucidate the nature of the imperative of healthcare delivery to which Canadians also inevitably subscribe, it would involve ferreting sometimes-cryptic fundamentals to shed light on seemingly benign assumptions inherent in our current practices. These assumptions are nonetheless, crucial to the conceptual leap required for the depth of understanding that all healthcare stakeholders need for the sustenance, relevance and continued quality control of our health systems.

Considering the significant role that health plays in the overall economy of any country, there is no doubt that we need to focus on the parameters significant to its evolution, in particular so that we could engineer them in our efforts to ensure the progress of our health services in the appropriate direction. This would mean taking the proper measures to facilitate the processes that result in the provision of qualitative healthcare delivery simultaneously reducing healthcare costs, hence spending. We would venture in this e-book to identify these measures, and to determine the most appropriate approaches to implementing them to assure the improvement in the quality of healthcare delivery in Canada, in both short and long terms.

Of Rights and Health

The agonizing probably ongoing in some quarters over recent developments in the pharmaceutical industry is reminiscent of the conflicts of rights that have emerged over the past several decades, and troubled many, the issues involved driven harder home more recently by Hillel Steiner, the renowned University of Manchester philosopher in his 1994 book[1], 'An Essay on Rights.' The implications of these conflicts for healthcare delivery are profound and complex, and would be even more so in the years ahead, as competing interests and pressures gel the essentially fluid mechanics of health services, into immutable yet transitory forms. December 10, 2006 marks another International Human Rights Day. The struggle to promote, protect, and preserve human rights continue worldwide. Yet, fifty-eight years after the United Nations adopted the Universal Declaration of Human Rights, questions remain regarding the status of the fundamental logic of rights in particular as a static or dynamic construct vis-à-vis its enduring applicability in an ever-changing world. When Pfizer Inc., announced on December 2, 2006 that it has stopped further trials of its experimental cholesterol medication torcetrapib, whose promise to increases the levels of the 'good' high-density lipoprotein (HDL) ushered hope to many, and potential sales boom to Pfizer substituting its top-selling Lipitor, which goes off patent in 2010, that the effects would boomerang was doubtless. Not only would the company have to contend with the loss of US$800 million in research and development (R&D) investment on torcetrapib, and the potential sales, $12.2 billion for Lipitor in 2005, it would lose, the company's shares fell $3.63, or 13%, to $24.23 in morning trading on December 4, 2006 on the New York Stock Exchange. This is not to mention the reported plans of the company to sell torcetrapib only in combination with Lipitor[2], which combined usage, resulted in the observed increased risk of death, and other complications, that incidentally aborted the trials. However, it is also not in doubt that the effects of torcetrapib's termination would rebound elsewhere across the pharmaceutical and health industries, and indeed, other industries, if not the economies within which Pfizer Inc., the world's largest drug maker operates. This underscores again, the salience of erstwhile philosophical discourses and even those ongoing, which illuminate the nature of the sorts of conflicts Steiner discussed eminently in his book. It is intuitive to expect the pharmaceutical industry to reflect on its current approach to drug development, for example, to consider the wisdom, or otherwise in investing hundreds of millions of dollars on R&D only to lose everything. Where such reflection leads the industry, puts the issue of the conflicts of rights squarely under the kliegs. Viewed in the contexts of the increasing paradigmatic shift in healthcare delivery toward the healthcare consumer being at the center-stage of the entire healthcare delivery enterprise, and what the drug industry in the U.S., for example, considers the increasing proclivity of health plans to dictate how much they intend to pay for medications, and indeed, the expectation becomes fact. What is more, R&D in the pharmaceutical industry appears to be struggling for viability, with just twenty medications receiving Food and Drug Administration (FDA) approval in 2005, versus thirty-six the year before, the

2005 R&D spending of almost US$40 billion, a 6% hike over spending in 2004, regardless. Questions regarding choices the pharmaceutical industry makes to enhance its performance and reduce costs, for example, focus on niche diseases fewer persons have, hence requiring smaller trials, or moving operations to other countries to slash costs, colliding with patients' rights, or are they interests, would certainly come up, and are in fact pertinent. This is more so, considering the potential adverse consequences of such choices on the quality of healthcare delivery, the effects of which if compromised would reverberate across all facets of healthcare delivery, including the pharmaceutical industry. The 'negative' rights envisioned in classical liberalism such as those to life, liberty, and property, or the 'pursuit of happiness' embody some of the 'positive' rights such as that to healthcare in the generic sense of the right to life. Would the right of the pharmaceutical industry to survive be clashing with those of individuals to life, of health systems to survive, as indeed, of economies, and would such a clash be as it is in conflict with the customary liberal notion of rights not to clash, be reason to question the viability of the basic logic of rights? The distinction between humans and things tangible or ephemeral is here moot, as the former constitutes the operational force of the latter, on the one hand, yet, are in being 'humans' distinct from them fundamentally. If we assumed that, there is a clash of rights between humans, as far as human operators made the choices the pharmaceutical industry makes, on behalf of investors and in whose interest the industry's survival counts, the effects of these choices impinging also on humans, some of who in fact might be investors in the industry, the question is apposite. Few would argue that rights should not guide each individual regarding actions allowed to avert conflicts between individuals or groups and to guarantee each individual's freedom, but contending that such conflicts are not in some instances, for example regarding healthcare, inevitable would likely be equally tenuous. Where for example would one draw the line between whose rights, that of the doctor, or of the patient, to consider superior to uphold, when the latter insists on receiving treatment for a chest disease that the latter refuses on the consideration that the treatment given the former continues to compromise ignoring advice on quitting an evidently unhealthy lifestyle? Such considerations rooted in this instance in clinical judgment also have significant economic underpinnings that could make adherents of utilitarianism whine, the association between humans, hard to impute as not inevitable and indeed, imperative, as recent world event in the health and other arena, clearly show. Furthermore, they raise critical questions about the significance of happiness, in Bethamistic pleasure/pain terms, pitching it against survival as the primal force of human motivation. This is particularly so as the logic of the avoidance of pain or the pursuit of pleasure inherent in certain acts such as an unhealthy lifestyle, despite full awareness, cognitively and emotionally, that is, of their consequences, for example, ill health seems oftentimes evidently cryptic. One could argue for an indirect, long-term, or chronic tendency toward suicide in some individuals that engage in such unhealthy lifestyles, but would such an argument not be internally inconsistent considering the option to terminate the said life more acutely were that indeed, the underlying motive for the unhealthy lifestyle? On the other hand, is it simply a matter of choice, in which case, is pain, the preference, or is pleasure equivalent to pain in some persons, and would this not put happiness as defined above in jeopardy? Should we therefore not be exploring survival, which even in obvious pain, seems to be the preferred state of human beings, as the rallying focus of human motivation? Would this not make it desirable therefore to have as Steiner counseled 'compossible,'[3] or mutually consistent rights, performable in tandem as our goal, while simultaneously acknowledging the potential, even the natural inclination of rights to clash in our individual pursuit of survival? Implicit in this formulation is the concept of competition, and paradoxically, and for it to work, that of collaboration, which both need no forcible gelling, being expedient to survival indeed, at all levels, individual, and corporate, and of health systems, even economies. Would the pharmaceutical industry then, in seeking solutions to its predicament, of the kind, for example, Pfizer is in, mentioned earlier, choose to adopt an approach wherein firms operate in smaller units, targeting niche diseases, and populations, as has Bristol-Myers, for example, which operates fewer research domains, now ten, from 35 just two years ago, be violating anyone's rights? Would it be ethico-morally wrong for the industry to exclude, as it invariably would, some individuals that have certain 'untargeted' diseases? Would such an atomistic approach to research and development in the pharmaceutical industry violate fundamental utilitarian principles, those of empathy versus antipathy, the moral injunction to seek the pleasure of the greatest number subordinated to seeking that of the fewer investors in the pharmaceutical industry? Should we construe the use by pharmaceutical companies of genetic biomarkers, for example, capable of predicting if a drug would be effective in a particular patient, to improve the efficiency and cost-effectiveness of clinical trials similarly or otherwise so long as the consequence is not atomistic? There are those that would consider the decision by pharmaceutical firms to operate in countries where labor is cheaper a violation of their rights to gainful employment, but is employment a right, or a privilege? Is it a benefit we have come to expect from some entity, in the public and private sector, or is it the duty of Pfizer to provide individuals with jobs in its home base, or for that matter anywhere else, and if not, why should we consider that it is infringing on the rights of anyone seeking its strategic goals? The flipside to this question is just as important, which is whether any firm has social responsibilities to where it operates, if indeed, there were no other justification for its 'duty' to make individuals in that locality otherwise happy creating and offering them jobs, preferring for example, a set of robots as its workforce. At the very least, it might be selling some of the products and services to the peoples, although as is the case in many of the developing countries where firms from America and Europe now seek cheap labor, most of the peoples, are struggling to earn enough to feed themselves and their families.

On the other hand, their struggles would likely not yield significant dividends were those that buy the products they make paying increasingly less for them due to dwindling disposable income, increasing competition among manufacturers, or sheer consumer-power, backed by enhanced knowledge of the pressure consumers could exert on prices in a free market economy. This would no doubt bounce back on corporate profitability, but would it be sufficient epiphany perhaps, of the inevitability of corporate social responsibility including not violating the rights of individuals to gainful employment, or put differently, contributing positively to the dynamics of the economy that avert job flights, if not actually creating and maintaining jobs? It is doubtful that any country would prefer the alternative of ever-increasing trade deficits with its potential catastrophic consequences not just for its economy, but also its very survival. In any case, it is just as unlikely that these firms would be particularly keen to engage in any activities that would essentially see their primary markets wither away, overtaken by other markets in the increasingly competitive global marketplace.

Thus, we see the need for a re-examination of the status of the logic of rights

to meet the exigencies of contemporary times. In other words, to focus more on the balance of rights, for example between privacy and free expression, rather than on the clash of rights, to see rights not as adversaries, but partners in an ongoing evaluation process of the survival of humankind that brings to the fore the very core of its existence, that of survival. That it has thus far performed creditably better than any other living being is why it has held such a central and pivotal position in what we could term appropriately, the earthly domain. Implicit in the ability to survive is that to be and to stay healthy, which underscores the significance of the developments in the pharmaceutical industry mentioned earlier, among others whose interplay continues to reveal the intricate pattern future healthcare delivery would dictate, then assume, only to dissolve, and compel new ones, in a perpetual inevitable motion toward progress. There is however, a proviso in this entire state of affairs, which the reason we cannot afford to ignore the necessity to re-conceptualize human rights to reflect our understanding of this inevitable motion, which otherwise could be a reversal of the gains humankind has so far made in the making, as old concepts fail miserably to address contemporary realities. How they could meet future challenges without such re-examination therefore, could only be conjectural. The point here is that the right to healthcare is the most fundamental of human rights, in keeping with the requirement for humankind to survive without which, even our earth will not, just as disuse results in the most elegant edifice crumbling ultimately, hence the need to address the crucial issues germane to ensuring this right. The question of such a right being natural or not is redundant, its enforceability in law, the underlying criterion for rights to be just that, the real, albeit debatable issue, in particular regarding the infringement of the right of others to healthcare, and indeed, to life, which are equally important reasons we should revisit the logic of rights. Could we and should we compel the pharmaceutical industry or firms in any other industry, to observe the rights of individuals to healthcare, for example by not restricting clinical trials to niche diseases, or by providing their employees stipulated health insurance coverage? Should we be even talking about rights without the legal means to enforce their observance? How would such legal constraints to provide healthcare work in healthcare delivery, for example, regarding the nature, type, and amount of health services provision by various health jurisdictions, vis-à-vis the limitations imposed by other constraints, the scarcity of healthcare resources, financial and manpower, for examples, and available institutional makeup? What role does the law, which alone restrains infringements on rights play in making these determinations, perhaps, via re-examining the fundamental logic of rights in the prevailing dispensation, as it in fact also influences that in the future? Yet, could such a role not interfere with other aspects of human activity in which legitimate claims to rights exist, the deprivation of which could compromise health, and the right to life? Would these considerations not lead us even if in a circuitous journey back via their potential implications for progress toward embracing democratic principles, which have so convincingly proven most capable of fostering the sort of balance of rights mentioned earlier, hence of ensuring the observance and enforcement of these rights? There is a sure contradiction suggested between liberty and rights, which in fact is fictitious, both fundamentally congruent, and essential to the realization of aspirations to each. The freedom of one individual predicates on that of the other, each not infringing on the other's rights, regardless of the competitive bent of either, indeed, as also earlier noted expressed in Steiner's concept of 'compossibility.' However, that rights could conflict does not mean there should be no rights, or flaw the concept, although striking the right balance between competing rights could become increasingly a chore with the proliferation of 'interests' masquerading as rights. In other words, should we accept the relativism of rights, and let them proliferate, subject rights to operational definitions free of incumbencies, or generate secondary from the primary, for example the right to basic health service as enshrined in the guiding principles of the Canada Health Act, for example, from that to healthcare, which we generated from that to life? Should we embrace this epigenetic structural approach, or adopt a functional one that, as we earlier noted, gels basic fluidity into tangible forms that being colloidal, could gel into others in keeping with contemporary realities, offering individuals the opportunities to continue to survive in a world whose changing parameters have the potential to make them moribund, otherwise? Is it therefore not appropriate for the Saskatchewan government not to introduce legislation that would enable it sue tobacco companies, as planned, with a view to recouping the amount it cost taxpayers to treat smoking-related diseases in the province, up to several million dollars yearly? Indeed, The Supreme Court of Canada has ruled that the Tobacco Damages and Health Care Costs Recovery Act, S.B.C. 2000, c. 30 is constitutionally valid, which created the avenue for British Columbia to sue tobacco firms for the expenses incurred treating smoking-related illnesses, British Columbia v. Imperial Tobacco Canada Ltd., 2005 SCC 49[4]. Should we consider legal restraints on a scientific endeavor that aims to breed a human and tortoise hybrid to discover the secrets of longevity, an infringement of the rights of the scientist, or not restraining the scientist that of the rest of us, or a particular individual that seeks legal redress feeling strongly so? Yet, the advance in knowledge both in the healthcare and technology, and indeed, other domains would likely create such situations in larger numbers in future, making the debate on rights and health, one in perpetuity, the need for easing the intellectual exercise this would spawn the reason for us to address the underlying logic of rights now. This is rather than an attempt at making life easier for those that would engage in this exercise in future, a practical necessity in any genuine efforts by any health jurisdiction not to infringe on the right to healthcare and hence to life of its residents. In other words, it is in consonance with efforts that any health jurisdiction would increasingly recognize are imperative, to meet the dual healthcare delivery objectives (DHDO) of the provision of qualitative health services simultaneously reducing health spending, which is inherent to the survival of any health system besides being crucial to meeting the rights of individuals to healthcare. Thus, even if we did not concur with health being a right, we are going to have to invoke, increasingly, the pressures that basic economic principles in an increasingly competitive global economic milieu impose on health services delivery in support of the need of individuals for qualitative healthcare. These needs, would eventually have to transition to rights, lest our health systems crumble, potentially taking with it other aspects of the economy. As noted with the case of liberty and rights earlier, these issues reveal the potential forces operating even in a free market economy to conflict, but not necessarily that they are incompatible, as indeed, they are not. What we need to do is sort out the differences our positions on the contradictions that emerge in dealing with any particular issue in an acrimonious-free debate that explores in-depth these issue and their potential ramifications, for the individual rights we are trying to establish. In other words, there is nothing a priori about rights, in a constantly changing world, the effect on which by the forces of change, natural, and manmade, expected, or not, could be as profound as not preparing to respond to an unknown virus that might emerge in a remote village somewhere, and spread around the world in days, killing millions. As with everything else in our world, and which is what it has always been, change makes the need for us to pay just as much attention to dynamic as we do to the static factors that drive our existence. We need to predicate the notion of rights on fundamental tenets whose essential feature is flexibility, or adaptability, in the more evolutionary sense in which this attribute has served humankind so well. It would be ominous for the future of health services, and the rights of individuals to life, therefore for a mentality of stagnation to permeate intellectual musings even in our homes, on such profound issues, as human rights, considering the tendency for the will of the peoples to prevail in the end. This makes coupling rights and health even more pragmatic, as the link, epigenetic, functional, or otherwise, is therein, quite evident. It is therefore likely that with the increasing consolidation of the central position of the healthcare consumer in healthcare delivery, would come, higher expectations of health services quality. Health systems would be under increasing pressure to deliver qualitative services on the one hand, and efficiently and cost-effectively, on the other, with pressures from healthcare consumers, and budgetary constraints, respectively, essentially choking. The link between rights and health would lead us for example to the potential consequences of not preventing the rapidly increasing epidemic of, for example, obesity, and diabetes, in many countries, on disease and economic burden, which even in countries with publicly funded health systems, we all have to bear.

Somewhere along the way would arise the issue of the right of an individual to eat even unhealthy food or not to exercise, to smoke cigarettes, even use street drugs, and drink large quantities of alcohol that some would pursue to its legal hilt to secure. Yet, others would insist that by not reining in these other individuals, for example, legislating against smoking, as is already the case, in most countries, where such laws exist, at least in public places, others could allege that society is allowing an infringement on their own rights. Even if tobacco had been around for centuries, we now have medical knowledge indicating its health risks, which would be foolhardy to ignore, considering the contemporary pressures on our health systems to say the least, to perform efficiently and cost-effectively, in favor to discountenance which not even the most passionate non-consequentialist would likely argue. This is considering the availability of objective evidence to buttress the appropriateness of the course of action toward achieving the overall consequences resulting from pursuing the achievement of the dual healthcare delivery objectives, for example. There is scientific research backing for one such course of action, for example, promoting the widespread implementation and utilization of healthcare information and communication technologies (healthcare ICT), in healthcare delivery. Research evidence also exists for a variety of other measures that health systems need to take to facilitate the achievement of the DHDO. Achieving the DHDO no doubt, helps ensure the rights of individuals to healthcare, hence to life, as they do the benefits of improved health of the populace to a country's economic growth and sustainable development. The nature of the link between rights and health systems would also become increasingly complex as the demand for meeting the requirements for the optimal expression of each becomes more urgent, yet more sophisticated, partly due to the phenomenal pace of the growth of knowledge in a variety of interlocking academic, technology, health, and other domains. In the healthcare delivery and healthcare information and communication technologies dyadic for example, the potential for the latter to enhance the right to life is increasingly bounteous as these technologies create enormous prospects for the delivery of qualitative health services.

It is instructive that despite the opportunities these technologies create in essentially achieving the dual healthcare delivery objectives, we are still not utilizing them enough in the delivery of health services in Canada. There is indeed, increasing research evidence of the potential benefits in health spending deploying these technologies in healthcare delivery pervasively for example, a study published in the September/October 2005 issue of the journal *Health Affairs*. This study estimated potential savings and costs of widespread diffusion of electronic medical record (EMR) systems and networking in the U.S., at US$81 billion annually[5]. It also noted that healthcare ICT-based chronic disease prevention and treatment could actually double those savings, other health, and social benefits accruing simultaneously. Indeed, the authors put the efficiency and safety savings of the pervasive implementation of interoperable EMR systems in that country at between US$142 and US$371 billion annually. Nonetheless, there is also no doubt about the hefty price tags of implementing these technologies, the Canadian government, for instance, which allotted $420 million in funding initially to implementing its national health information networks, now billed to spend $1.2 billion[6]. Should we not in fact therefore weigh these considerations appropriately to determine if the latter would outweigh the former, and vice versa? Would the benefits derivable from the initial investments in these technologies, even if in the long term, and even considering the total costs of ownership (TCO) not far outweigh these upfront costs? Would we not in fact be infringing on the rights of Canadians not investing in these technologies, and not promoting their widespread adoption by healthcare providers, and indeed, other healthcare stakeholders, including the healthcare consumer? Could we not argue that this is in fact the case considering the right of Canadians to life the most fundamental as we noted earlier? There are in fact compelling reasons besides the moral dimensions implied in the right to life foundation for the provision of qualitative health services by the country's health systems to all its peoples, as indeed, enshrined in the Canada Health Act, as would become apparent as we proceed in our discussion here. Thus, it is ironical that Canada, which started on its nationwide health information networks, back in 1997 and plans to have electronic health records (EHR), for 50% of its population by 2010 still lags behind many comparable industrialized countries in the deployment of these networks in healthcare delivery. Germany for example, was the first Organization for Economic Cooperation and Development (OECD) country to start investing in healthcare ICT. Starting in 1993, it plans to complete in 2006, its national health information network, which would encompass, 'smart card' technology. The United Kingdom (U.K) spends substantially more than we do on its network program, which although started in 2002, is the costliest and most inclusive worldwide the goal, to have an interlinked healthcare record, e-appointment and prescription systems, and a nationwide health information network accessible to all its doctors and other healthcare providers by 2014[6]. Estimate of total investment as of 2005 are US$1.0 billion, US$1.8 billion and US$11.5 billion, for Canada, Germany and the U.K., respectively, that for the U.S., US$ 125 million[6], total investments per capita for the same countries, US$1.85, US$21.20, US$192.79, and US$0.43, respectively, and for the same year. Canada and the U.S are also among the countries in the OECD that the 2006 Commonwealth Fund/Harris Interactive survey that included over 6,000 primary care physicians (PCPs) in Australia, Canada, Germany, the Netherlands, New Zealand, the United Kingdom, and the United States, including over 1,000 U.S. physicians, showed utilized healthcare ICT the least[7]. Just 23% of Canadian doctors reported the use of electronic medical records (EMRs), 28% of U.S. doctors, versus 98%, 92%, 89%, and 79%, of physicians in the

Netherlands, New Zealand, the U.K., and Australia, respectively[7]. The survey also showed that Canadian and U.S. doctors are also unlikelier to have decision support systems (DSS) such as computer alerts regarding drug interactions for example, 10% and 23%, respectively, versus 93%, and 40% in the Netherlands, and Germany, respectively, for example. Additionally, 40% of Canadian and U.S doctors reported difficulty identifying patients past due for a test or preventive care, versus 20% or less that did doctors from the other countries. Considering the importance of primary care in the healthcare delivery process, being the entry-point in most cases of the pathways to care, and the importance of PCPs to primary care, should we not consistent with global initiatives to improve the quality and performance of health systems, enunciate policies to boost the efficiency and efficacy of primary care in Canada? Would formulating such policies for example on the widespread implementation and use of healthcare ICT, not be in keeping with our commitment to the right of Canadians to life, with the technologies able to help improve access to care, doctors diagnose and treat patients better, and improve patient safety, reducing medical errors? In fact, not many would likely dispute that we need to start to offer healthcare providers financial incentives for qualitative service provision, including the implementation and utilization of healthcare ICT, and among others. In the U.K., for example, up to 95% of doctors receive such incentives including for enhanced value proposition such as the provision of preventive services, and the management of chronic diseases, in both of which healthcare ICT could no doubt play a significant role. As noted earlier, there are many crucial reasons adducible for the need to ensure the delivery of qualitative health services, besides the moral reasons against not so doing, one being pecuniary, predicated on basic economic principles, for examples the fundamental and inevitable scarcity of resources, and the need for their astute management resulting thereof. Interestingly, the roots and potential consequences of these economic principles coincide with the underlying foundations of the logic of rights, in particular the assumptions behind some of its more recent flavors. The question arises in this context, why we should concern ourselves with providing or not, all the needs of everyone in the first place, as though they were their rights. A related question would be why we need to allocate and manage resources efficiently and cost-effectively. Does government have some sort of atavistic contractual obligation to do so and would we be trampling on anyone's rights not so doing for example? It is plausible that the varying expression of the desire by some to appropriate whatever is available by whatever means to fulfill even their most trivial requirement that could create potentially chaotic situations has to do with this tendency to worry about scarcity. On the other hand, it might be evolutionarily shrewd to give this expression free reign while simultaneously curtailing it under different circumstances, in communal appropriation in the former case for example, and in the moderation of individual aspirations in the latter. The link between this differential approach to our potential penchant for ascribing attributes both profound and mundane to ourselves and to ours reveals a crucial aspect of the logic of rights whose manifest expression contracts sharply with its intrinsic worth. Should we, based on the differential treatment given the expression of desire, and indeed, motive, mentioned above, not wonder what the ultimate desire in either instance is, and is it not essentially self-preservation? Is it not therefore imperative that we embrace the basic economic principles mentioned above, considering our desire for self-preservation, but does it make the latter therefore a right imbued with universal truth, a moral universalism without any social, political, or historical antecedents or encumbrances? That we have a tendency to strive to survive and that our ability to survive depend in large measure on that of ourselves in association with others, to maximize the opportunities available to us in so doing, subordinating our individual needs at times, to collective needs, in a suave expression of the logic of rights to which we must subscribe. Thus, the fundamental individual quest for survival intertwined with that of the group makes the mandate of the group therefore to ensure the survival of its individuals, in other words the right of its individuals to life. Put differently, the survival of each individual depends on that of the group and that of the group, on the individuals therein. In contemporary times, the associations mentioned above often transcend the ethnic or cultural, social, economic, and geopolitical interests, key determinants in a world where resources are even scarcer with continuous depletion over the millennia. Even countries therefore must continue to ponder over the precise loci of their best interests in the global scheme of things. These considerations are apposite in any, regarding the key role of healthcare delivery in the unraveling of the newer meanings ascribable to the rights and the understanding of its logic. There is no doubt that in the current dispensation, with sovereign states the default oversight mechanism for ensuring the validity of the concept of rights, that rights do what they ought to do, the question of whether or not they do so is moot. This is because many such states clearly not only do not with regard even the internationally agreed rights, but flagrantly do the opposite, flout them. It would seem that this is a simple matter, which paradoxically it is as we would soon explain, but it is uncertain that such states have a fundamental grasp of the logic of rights, essentially that rights are self-enforcers, ultimately. In other words, as much as we might invoke legal authority in enforcing mutually agreed rights, including at the inter-governmental level of, for example, imposing sanctions on the aberrant state, that such measures hardly redeem them attests to the paradox mentioned earlier. This paradox is that of one simple measure, sanctions, ineffective, another, the inevitable process of change that the expression of the collective, rooted in the individual, tendency to survive, which is self-enforced, working. The collapse of the Soviet state, the economic revival of China, and the consequences of every tendency toward protectionism, even in the Western world, among others are testimonies to this process.

That rights do not therefore need legal teeth at the conceptual level is evident, although at the practical level, would be, as in other spheres of our endeavors, the need for law and other, if only to preempt the potential of disruptive elements, natural and artificial to delay progress that is inevitable, anyway, either way. This last point is also crucial, as we have seen in history the collective will induced by a variety of means, for example, in Jonestown, Guyana, not too long ago, expressed in the morbid direction. Similarly, we, as humans could collectively will ourselves as a group to extinction, or indeed, so willed, by our actions, in for example, not preserving or actively damaging the environment, or by natural catastrophes, caught literally flat-footed. It is clear from the foregoing therefore, that we assert our rights to life based on it being crucial to the survival of others and to that of us all as humans. It might seem at first oversimplified to consider that what happens to one person, for example, trampling on the right of that person to life, crucial to the survival of humankind, but we have seen in history the tyranny unleashed on millions by one deranged individual that happened to assume a leadership position in a group, or country. This is not suggesting that anyone trampled on the right to life of those tyrants, although had some of them, who might have clearly had some form of mental illness had availed themselves of treatment, things might have gone differently. This underscores the conflict of rights mentioned earlier, which in fact, is why the logic of rights sometimes is questionable. Is the tendency of some to will themselves in the morbid direction, or be so-willed, enough reason for trampling on the rights of others to life? These considerations also bring to the fore, the issues of the conceptual and practical challenges in dealing with rights. For example, to what extent should, the others whose rights, an individual with some form of mental illness, would perhaps trample upon hacking them to death or even maiming them, driven by chronic persecutory delusions, be accountable for not somehow, ensuring that the individual receives treatment? Should we simply leave him or her alone if not interested in receiving treatment, or because we could not enforce treatment so as not to violate his/her right? Could matters have gone differently had we offered treatment earlier, before the condition became chronic, or had we in fact prevented, if possible the condition, for example, the use by an individual of Crystal Meth, which could present with schizophrenia-like symptoms, including persecutory delusions? It is evident that the right to life should, as proposed earlier, therefore be contingent conceptually, with practical legal trappings, acknowledging its roots in the tendency for survival an imperative for collaboration. The tendency of the group to survive bestows the right to life, in a manner of speaking as opposed to the biological tendency to survive per se so doing, as even if it consumed itself, that life would not last very long, conducted solo. Is it any wonder then that there is hardly if any only survivor of a species of living things? What we propose here is a functional, cross-linked approach to the issue of rights, including the right to life, and by extension, to healthcare delivery in Canada. The real issues regarding rights should be what the consequences for the survival of an individual, or individuals that have a certain disease condition, would be consequent upon the measures taken in the pharmaceutical industry for example to reduce costs. In other words, the practical aspects of the right to life are even more crucial than its conceptual roots in protecting it and ensuring its observance. In this regard, the provision of health for all is an important component of securing these conceptual roots, in other words, what really ensuring the right to life is all about. What are the implications of these issues for the provision of qualitative health services to Canadians? In the first place, they confirm the wisdom in the lofty ideals of the health system of Canada, embodied in the Canada health Act, although it is another matter what we should do with the health system in the years ahead. Simply based on what we have discussed thus far, it is clear that no health system could afford to be static lest it fails to meet its mandate of ensuring the preservation of Canadians' right to life. It is in fact the case that no health system is perfect, or could ever be perfect, hence the need for a constant reappraisal of the system with a view to improving it and making it able to meet this mandate. It is unlikely that a health system would be perfect because of not just the changes inherent in the system, which time for example, imposes, with respect, say of a particular structure, for example, its building, almost a century old that just does not suit the current practice of medicine for a variety of reasons. An inherent factor could also be changing practice due to new medical knowledge, not to mention those imposed from without, due to developments in other fields, such as healthcare ICT, accounting, economic, management, even changes in the political and social milieu. Any health system that is unresponsive to these changes would invariably compromise itself, the sort of 'willing in the morbid direction' mentioned above, hence the need or in fact the imperative of the Canadian health system to undergo continuing change. It has to be adaptable, and to be able to respond effectively to the likely harsh realities it might face in the years ahead resulting from population aging, among others. We should for example, in promoting the widespread adoption and use of healthcare ICT recognize the need to involve doctors, as the U.K., and Australia, for example did, identifying early adopters and utilizing them to convince fellow doctors of the need for and the benefits of healthcare ICT. Many believe that such measures helped boost the implementation of the technologies in these countries, and indeed, we should, as noted earlier, even introduce incentives that would further encourage doctors and other healthcare providers to implement the technologies. The Australian government in the late 1990s gave GPs financial incentives to implement computers and clinical software packages for prescribing drugs and patient health data/information communication and sharing, an effort deemed partly responsible for more widespread computer use by GPs, from 15% to 70% in 1997 and 2000, respectively. Indeed, the findings of a recent survey indicated that Australia has been able to achieve its significant progress in healthcare ICT adoption, partly because of the use of financial incentives and other government programs[8]. The survey showed that 98% of 3,000 GPs surveyed, 1,186 or 40% of which replied, used clinical software systems for regular e-prescribing, 94%, to update medication lists, 88% to check for drug-drug interactions, and 87% to monitor medication allergies (87%). Seventy percent of the doctors used software to check drug-disease interactions, and 65%, to record their reasons for prescribing certain medications. Many of the Australian GPs said that they used a clinical software package as electronic health records, 85% used it to order laboratory tests, 84% to update patient allergy data, and equal number, to generate patient health summaries, fewer doctors using it to develop and update disease management plans, record progress notes, access patients' educational material, and for clinical audits. In the above study, over 50% of the GPs acknowledged receiving a Practices Incentives Program payment, the Australian government gave primary care doctors to encourage the adoption of electronic medical records (EMR), another 32%, a Broadband for Health incentive payment for the implementation and use of high speed Internet. Incidentally, the survey also showed that just 58% of the GPs used the software package to generate patient lists, a key tool for chronic diseases management, and many did not use the e-DSS functions of the software package in consultations, for example to review prescribing data/information, patients' risk factors, or chronic disease guidelines. These features, which only about 20% of the GPs use, could reduce medical errors significantly, hence enhance patient enhance, and improve overall care quality. Indeed, it is unlikely that we could derive full benefits from healthcare ICT not utilizing its full features, another key aspect of the considerations regarding upfront investments in these technologies, vis-à-vis their overall long-term benefits. Considering the expected increase in the prevalence of chronic conditions in the country, it is no doubt important that we are cognizant of such developments in Australia that have made the country's GPs achieve universal utilization of electronic medical records (EMRs) in less than a decade. We should also note the areas needing improvement, specifically the use of software functionalities that would help improve the management of chronic diseases, among others, for example, the interoperability of these technologies, the issue of standards, and other technical, legal, and other issues. Indeed, we should take a cue from other countries too. For example, regarding privacy concerns, we could learn much from the measures that other countries have taken regarding stipulating standards for patient data/information collection, usage, and disclosure. The relatively slow pace of the widespread use of healthcare information and communication technologies in healthcare delivery in Canada reflects difficulties with some of the technical and privacy issues problems mentioned above, but also indicates problems with the health systems in the countries, which are essentially under provincial and territorial jurisdictions. These systems issues are varied and many, some common to all and others peculiar to certain of these jurisdictions. Nonetheless, we need to address the issues to ensure that we do nothing that could compromise the right to life of Canadians and indeed, the collective desire of Canadians to survive as an entity. One cannot gainsay the need symbiotic dyadic between the individual and the group, and the right to life, both need and for which both need each other. In the 1990s in the U.S., healthcare delivery came under the increasing influence of investors and investor-owned companies, many hospitals, nursing homes, home care services, and health maintenance organizations (HMOs), transitioned to for-profit firms, drug companies, diagnostic services, medical devices and health insurance firms, all waxed stronger. This emergence of the medical- industrial complex, Arnold Relman, former Editor of *The New England Journal of Medicine*, foreshadowed in 1980, noting its potential to creates overuse and service fragmentation, cautioning the need to put public interests before stockholders'[9]. His concerns about overemphasis on technology was apt in some respects, in particular if these technologies were used incorrectly, defensively, as in their use just so the physician avoids litigation, and irrationally, for examples, which besides adding perhaps adding little if anything to diagnostic or treatment efficacy increases avoidable costs. The use of healthcare ICT in Canada would no doubt need to avoid these problems, some of them more likely to arise than even in the U.S., because of the moral hazard inherent in universal healthcare delivery systems, such as ours. In other words, the tendency not to take the necessary care in preventing illness, or to utilize services more than necessary, among variants because they are free, could escalate costs, in particular with the use or overuse of expensive technologies such as the CT scanner. Yet we do not want to seem to place reduction in health spending over and above the right of Canadians to life. It would therefore be necessary for each health jurisdiction to explore the modus for achieving the right balance between these competing issues, which underscores the point made earlier about the need for a balance rather than a clash of rights. It also highlights the reason for the emphasis we have thus far placed on promoting the widespread adoption and implementation of healthcare ICT in the country, because these technologies could help us achieve the dual healthcare delivery objectives (DHDO), namely the provision of qualitative health services to Canadians, simultaneously reducing health spending.

Should we envisage the emergence of a medical-industrial complex here in

Canada able to, and in addition to some of the cautions Relman mentioned, have considerable influence on health policy formulation and implementation in the country, seeking the interests of stakeholders, at the expense of those of the rest of us? This question highlights some of the potential issues our health system would confront in the years ahead, given the simmering debate over whether the country should have a parallel private health system. It is inconceivable that interest groups would not continue to exert pressure on government as indeed, already exists, and some of these groups are in the health industry. The point in fact is that the operations of these various groups constitute, along with the interplay of a variety of other associations, the functional elements of a vibrant democracy and need encouraged, in keeping with the need to promote a balance of rights and discourage their conflict. It seems unlikely though that we could determine the relative influence of any group with certainty as this depends on the closeness of its components to the interest area in government or whichever locale it lies, which would of course vary, with a change of government for example. The important point then is to have the required mechanisms in place to ensure the smooth operations of these interactive forces, without anyone's right to life placed in jeopardy. It is necessary to observe here though that even if the intensity of the influence of these groups matched that of those in the U.S., which Relman cautioned against, but which indeed, occurred and which some blame for some of the woes of the country's health systems currently, should we worry overly about it compromising our health system, perhaps significantly? No doubt we should if it could but could it? To the extent that the bulk of our healthcare Medicare funds, this would be difficult as the intensity of competition within the health system is minimal mostly not manifest as vicious competition, the sort encountered sometimes, in the private sector, but competition it is nonetheless, to the extent that a particular health system could benchmark itself for its strategic intent. The truth of the matter though is that not only would it not be enough to attempt in each budgetary year to outsmart itself, health systems might soon need to actually generate funds to fund itself, or at least some of its programs, developing innovative approaches to healthcare delivery. This does not necessarily mean its clinical dimension, but in a generic sense, the overall series of processes that culminate in the healthcare delivery enterprise. Would it not be smarter for the chief executive of a health region A, whose service unit B is essentially redundant as clientele dropped for a variety of reasons, to 'outsource' it to health region B that has valid economic reasons to keep providing the services? Could the implementation of the necessary telehealth technologies, not make access still possible for the few that still need the services, for example, rather than having a full-time specialist wait around without seeing any patient all day? Could the chief executive A not invest the money saved in some other service area or even in ventures that could generate money for the health region, for example, a cafeteria for visiting patients' relatives and friends, in addition to the convenience to these peoples and the boost to the hospital's public image? Were these health jurisdictions to compete with a parallel health system, though, the competition would intensify drastically, the potential hegemony of a medical-industrial complex likelier to manifest stronger. This explains in part why some oppose the idea of a parallel private health system, apprehensive of the potential depletion of already scarce resources in the public health system, worsening its existential problems in some instances. Yet, the question would arise again, how likely these developments would violate the rights of Canadians to life. Again, we should be measured in our apprehension, avoiding any tendency to catastrophize what some would consider benign, perhaps even something that protects, and preserves the peoples' right to life, in particular rights viewed conceptually, so long as the necessary institutions exist to ensure that in assuring the right of the overall group, those of its individuals' remain viable. In other words, it is possible to view the activities of this medical-industrial complex as eventually and overall favorable for the perpetuation of society, as they keep economic activities and market forces operational, which are ingredients of economic buoyancy. Whereas if somehow, they made health services too costly and beyond the reach of Canadians, not only would they be infringing on the right of the peoples to life, their overall, albeit long-term, effect on the economy and the market, negative, which would adversely affect this complex too. This was why we wondered earlier if it could have similar effects as with the concerns Relman raised mentioned earlier, and why perhaps, the complex could not be the only, if not in fact, not the main reason, that the U.S. health system has the problems it does currently. In keeping with the idea that rights are self-enforced, even such complexes would eventually modulate themselves, regardless of the system, political or economic in which they exist. The point here is that rights all would emanate from that to life, including to healthcare delivery. The evolution of these rights is inevitable as change also is, our new realities necessitating key adaptation to continue to survive let alone thrive. We in Canada need to recognize and accept these facts, adapting our health system to meet the needs of our changing times. We could still operate within the ambit of the universal health services delivery whose five critical principles the Canada Health Act embodies. However, we would need to reorient ourselves and determine the means by which we could continue to enjoy the qualitative health services to which we are accustomed. One key aspect of this is to recognize the need to achieve the dual healthcare delivery objectives (DHDO) as a crucial component of our quest to ensure that our individual rights to life remain intact, and that we are also able to survive as a country. In enabling, us to achieve the DHDO, healthcare information and communication technologies become key players in our health systems. Hence, another key aspect of the reorientation is that of accepting the need to promote the widespread implementation and use of these technologies in healthcare delivery. It is therefore necessary for us to erase the legacy of the sort of findings the 2006 Commonwealth Fund/Harris Interactive survey earlier mentioned. We need to take the issue of healthcare ICT more seriously. Indeed, we need to recognize the need to have qualitative, shared, accessible data and information in all aspects of societal functioning, to ensure responsive and accountable policy formulation and decision-making, regardless of domain, or its level. This need ties closely with that to rectify information asymmetry, what some would consider the bane of patient-centered healthcare delivery, the type any health system, including the Canadian health system would increasingly embrace inevitably, in the coming years, as part of its efforts to achieve the DHDO. Thus, health systems, including ours in Canada, would have little if any choice to provide information, needed for such decision making, to all healthcare stakeholders, or create the enabling environment for its provision. Such provision, being a transaction would have costs implications, which again, as part of the goals of the information provision in the first place, we would attempt to slash, necessitating the provision of this information efficiently, and cost-effectively, which again, underlines the pervasiveness of the role of information and communication technologies in other domains too. In other words, these technologies are the key integrators and facilitators of our modern existence, and indeed, as they are for healthcare delivery, veritable yardstick for measuring progress including that of healthcare delivery, and indeed, of society as a whole. It is in keeping with our appreciation of the right to life of Canadians therefore that all health jurisdictions redouble their efforts in implementing healthcare ICT. There needs to be coordination at all levels of government of the various efforts already made and that we continue to make, which though could be counterproductive and wasteful, otherwise. This would be precisely the case, were the legacy systems of hospitals, family doctors, physician groups, health centers, and community health services, among others, to remain in 'silos' as they mostly currently are, the communication and sharing of patient information even among healthcare providers within the same town or city, essentially difficult if not impossible electronically. It doubtful that anyone would argue that we have maximized the potential of the huge investments in these technologies that we have so far made considering the results of the 2006 Commonwealth Fund/Harris Interactive survey mentioned earlier, for example. Meantime, the country not only continues to spend increasing amounts of its resources on healthcare delivery, the potential for these investments yielding maximum benefits not realized, arguable, even if we disregarded the likely costs in disease burden, the resources we could have saved, and reallocated to other needy areas, we could not, potentially compromising the right of someone to life.

The issue of rights therefore implies the compelling duty to ensure the efficient and cost-effective operations of our many systems, health and others. This is the self-enforcement principle mentioned earlier that is inherent in rights, which makes its legal enforcement, at least at the conceptual level unnecessary, and at the practical level only pragmatic. This pragmatic aspect is a major cause of controversy in some instances, admittedly, for example, regarding the right to death, that of individuals to will themselves in the morbid direction as we noted earlier. This is why the role of the state in ensuring the right to life is only indirect, as it might as well be ensuring the right to death, the self-enforcing principle, which is direct, still going to take its course. This means there is not much anyone could do to stop a group, society, or country, which has willed itself in the morbid direction, and that only that group could redirect itself. Every group, hence individual is therefore ultimately struggling to find the balance of rights that would ensure its survival, which conventional wisdom would suggest is the commoner than its demise, which we have seen some groups or countries seemingly do even in contemporary times, some even to take others, willing and unwilling along with them on their moribund path. Just as history tells us, therefore, we in Canada must develop and manage all our resources most judiciously, in healthcare delivery for example, not ignoring the potential benefit of healthcare ICT in helping us achieve the DHDO, to be able to survive. We would certainly need these resources in negotiating and forging the necessary alliances crucial in determining the right balance that would not only secure, but preserve the rights of Canadians to life, and by extension that of the country. This no doubt is the will of the overwhelming majority of Canadians.

References

1. Steiner, Hillel An Essay on Rights. Oxford: Blackwell, 1995.

2. Available at: http://www.nytimes.com/2005/03/07/business/07pfizer.html?ex=1267851600&en=ba1e0b3d1500b69e&ei=5088&partner=rssnyt Accessed on December 10, 2006

3. Available at: http://www.cato.org/pubs/journal/cj15n2-3-14.html Accessed on December 10, 2006

4. Available at: http://www.lawsociety.sk.ca/newlook/Archive/Archive05Sep.htm Accessed on December 10, 2006

5. Hillestad, Richard; Bigelow, James; Bower, Anthony; Girosi, Federico; Meili, Robin; Scoville, Richard; Taylor, Roger. *Health Affairs*, Sep/Oct2005, Vol. 24 Issue 5, p1103-1117, 15p; DOI: 10.1377/hlthaff.24.5.1103; (*AN 18282540*)

6. Anderson, G.F., Frogner, B.K., Johns, R.A., and Reinhardt, U.E., Health Care Spending and Use of Information Technology in OECD Countries, *Health Affairs*, May/June 2006 25(3):819-31

7. Schoen, C., Osborn, R., Trang Huynh, P., Doty, M., Peugh, J., and Zapert, K., On The Front Lines of Care: Primary Care Doctors' Office Systems, Experiences, and Views in Seven Countries, *Health Affairs* Web Exclusive (Nov. 2, 2006):w555-w571.

8. McInnes, D.K., Saltman, D.C., Kidd, M.R., General Practitioners' Use of Computers for Prescribing and Electronic Health Records, *Medical Journal of Australia*, July 17, 2006 185(2):188-91

9. Relman AS. The new medical-industrial complex. N Engl J Med 1980; 303: 963-70.

On the Mimicry of a Lamb

Changes in economic forces taken together influence the outcome of elections[1]. These macroeconomic variables thus affect human behavior, hence would, in theory affect human well-being, including happiness, which research has confirmed, changes in reported well-being correlated with those in macroeconomic variables for example, gross domestic product (GDP)[2]. There is also research evidence of the huge psychological costs of cyclical economic downturns, in a year, potentially much more than the GDP cost of a year of recession[2], costs with which we would have little if any choice but to start to reckon in our computations of the cost of cyclical downturns in the prevailing dispensation. Intuitively, it is reasonable to say that we have the potential to work harder and be more productive when we are healthy, and happy. Yet, the exact nature and extent of the link between happiness/well-being and economic fluctuations remains controversial. Even with the Keynesian/real-business-cycle wrangle, regarding the extent of the effects of macroeconomic variations sidestepped, the viewpoint of the former regarding recessions being costly disruptions to a country's economic organization, or of the latter that we not as Keynesians overestimate the costs of business cycle downturns, but consider them desirable corrections to productivity setbacks, disregarded, its significance is evident. This is that we need alternative ways to evaluate the costs of economic downturns, a purpose that focus on well-being and happiness would serve creditably. It is also an exercise that would likely enable us appreciate the closer affinity of happiness to the concept of experienced utility, with its accent on the delight obtained from consumption[3,4], as opposed to the decision utility of customary economic theory, which stresses choice being simply indicative of preference. No doubt, that the choices politicians make, predicated not surprisingly on their chances of being re-elected, assumed from perceived or established electorate satisfaction with the status quo, sway unemployment, inflation, GDP per capita, and other variables, underscores the importance of the difficulty, hence controversy over, making a direct correlation between happiness and macroeconomic variables. This is more so, specifically regarding the direction of the motion between the two, at a reference point in time. Yet, the experiential element pervades any consideration of either, and as the study mentioned earlier indicated, with the immense psychological costs of an economic recession, far more than its effects on the fall in GDP, and rise in unemployment, with the potential to further escalate health spending, and worsen the economy, well-being/happiness, indeed, health in general, becomes pivotal consideration. In other words, increasing attention to the macroeconomics of health would become necessary as our understanding of the consequences of the interplay between the various elements of the health and macroeconomic dyadic for healthcare delivery on the one hand, and for economic growth and sustainable development on the other, improves. Meantime, there is no gainsaying the ubiquity of the ramifications of the dyadic on health systems, even as efforts to decompose it continue apace, for example manifest in the soothing effect of the welfare state on the psychological, hence disease burden of recession with the association between higher unemployment benefits and improved national well-being. Back in the early 2000s, when the UK government revealed its plan to double health spending over ten years to more than £120 billion, up to a maximum of £184 billion by 2022, many saw it as a throwback to vintage Labor strategy of placing social justice above business, others a restatement of the country's universal access to care doctrine[5]. However, few considered the plan a commitment to the contemporary international macroeconomic zeitgeist, a novel worldwide orthodoxy on health rooted in the report of the Commission on Macroeconomics and Health that Jeffrey Sachs headed. The report, released in December 2001, considered investing in health the most effective way to eliminate poverty in low and middle-income countries, a finding the plan's critics did not think the U.K. government ought to have applied to an industrialized economy. The Sachs Commission also recommended the establishment by each country, of a National Commission on Macroeconomics and Health to coordinate the increase in health investment. Also in the U.K., the Wanless Report, which the Chancellor of the Exchequer commissioned and that constitutes the centerpiece of the Chancellor's National Health Service (NHS) strategy, noted the importance of public engagement with health in any effort to reform the NHS, whose success would increasingly depend more on patients' attitude and behavior than on the services provided. Thus, engaged healthcare consumers would likelier embrace disease prevention initiatives, for example, or participate more actively in decision making regarding their health, which would improve service delivery, reduce disease prevalence, hence healthcare costs, and ultimately, health spending. With the U.K., therefore spending less on healthcare delivery, at the same providing improved care, it is doubtful that the potential positive effects on macroeconomic variables of these developments would be contestable. The corollary is therefore likely to be true, which makes it reasonable, if not in fact mandatory to acknowledge that the seemingly benign expression of the association between macroeconomic and health variables in industrialized countries, belies the potential for catastrophe ignoring this link anywhere in the world could spawn, which might explain the Chancellor's inclination not to so do. This is why it is also unlikely for example to ignore the increasing percentage of the GDP many of these countries currently spend on health, not to mention changing demographics and other factors that threaten current approaches to health services delivery, including funding, with potential spill-over effects on other aspects of the economy, for examples, pensions, and social welfare. Pressure due to geopolitical alliances resulting in for example, changes in migration patterns, are also crucial players in the dynamics of health services provision, which could compromise, or otherwise, the interplay of a country's health and macroeconomic variables. It would increasingly become necessary therefore, for countries and health jurisdictions to seek ways by which they would delivery qualitative health services, cost-effectively and efficiently. A key aspect of this would be relocating the healthcare consumer at the epicenter of the healthcare delivery shakeup. Part of the changes the healthcare consumer would need to undergo would predicate on the requirements for the provision of higher quality services, including more transparency and accountability in the conduct of the healthcare delivery process. This implies rectifying the information asymmetry that currently plagues the health sector, ensuring that the healthcare consumer no longer lacks crucial information for rational decision making for example, regarding health matters. Thus, that information communication and sharing would need to be bidirectional is a proviso for enhanced services to the healthcare consumer implies the latter's active involvement in making this happen, efficiently and cost-effectively, including investing in the required healthcare care information and communication technologies (ICT). Future health systems would therefore need to court, actively, health services end-users to complete the chain of information communication and sharing essential for the achievement of the DHDO, more so considering the enormous financially outlay of many developed countries in these technologies, which researches have shown have the potential to achieve these twin goals. Another aspect of the involvement of health services end users is attitudinal change, to inculcate the need to accept responsibilities being the flipside of rights in the healthcare delivery enterprise in the healthcare consumer, so for example, to reduce the rates of missed appointments, which could be crucial to reducing wait times, for instance, for other end users. Indeed, in general, it would be necessary for health jurisdictions to promote responsible use of health services, which again underscores the need to invest in healthcare ICT, technologies that could help with appointment scheduling and rescheduling. Healthcare ICT could also assist in reducing practice mistakes, including medication errors, and by making relevant information available in real time at the point of care, further help improve patient safety, and the overall quality of care, which underlines the need to promote the use of these technologies among another group of healthcare stakeholders, the healthcare providers. Indeed, the essential basis for the maximization of the opportunities that healthcare ICT offer in enhancing the contribution of healthcare delivery to the health and macroeconomic dyadic is the effective and efficient operations of a network of interoperable information and communication systems that enable, and facilitate multi-level data and information sharing. In other words, we cannot assume that we have achieved this goal or that we have optimized the resources we have in so doing, without the patient information-communication chain linked and the cycle completed. There are no doubt about challenges surfacing along the way in the widespread adoption of these technologies, for example, embedding decision-support tools into electronic health record systems (EHR), resolving standards issues, and ensuring interoperability. This means that our efforts in promoting the widespread adoption of these technologies must be ongoing, lest we lose valuable time in maintaining the integrity of the dyadic, creating avenues for prospective setbacks, the consequences of which on not just the health and well-being of individuals, but also on overall national economic prosperity, potentially immense.

It seems from the foregoing that we need to pay more attention to ensuring health service delivery meets certain important goals, and that the healthcare consumer is at the center of the issues involved in so doing. Indeed, policy debates regarding not just health, but also other domains of a country's economy, for instance, social services, public health, transportation, family services, and the environment, are increasingly concerned with the use of subjective indicators of well-and ill-being as drivers of policy, at local, and national levels, along with and different from social and economic indicators. Subjective well-being as we noted earlier has close bearings to fluctuations in macroeconomic variables, hence a country's economic prosperity. It is therefore important, as part of our efforts to improve health services to be, cognizant of the concerns, and well-being of the citizenry, which is an essential constituent of a democratic society anyway, but engaging in which could provide valuable data and information that could influence new policy formulation and changes to the existing ones. Concerns over particular aspects of healthcare delivery could help reveal problems, and in identifying the solutions to them. This could result in improved service provision that could help overall improve the well-being and happiness of service recipients, with positive consequences for not just these recipients, but for the entire country. Even without specific concerns lodged, it is in the interests of health jurisdictions to seek to alleviate if not prevent demoralization, depression, misery, and other negative psychological states, to prevent the negative cumulative effects they would necessarily have that could, as noted earlier, compromise the country's economic prosperity. This is besides creating potentially avoidable, or at least treatable diseases, and their burden, in material, and intangible terms, neither of which would augur well for their interests and those of their families in the short and long terms. The seemingly simple assessments of life satisfaction and happiness for example, and indeed, more specific indicators such as mood, perceived psychological and physical health, subjective of time availability and use, among others, in surveys conducted at all levels of a health jurisdiction, on large samples to sharpen interpretation, including trends. They could also facilitate the ability to generalize their findings could provide valuable information with far-reaching health and economic implications for a country. We should indeed then conduct these surveys periodically, with psychometrically-valid instruments, targeting specific groups, on short and long term bases, using indicators sensitive to changes in subjective well-being, hence modifiable by policy changes, whose effects we should also endeavor to measure, to gauge their effectiveness and the need or otherwise to implement new policies. The importance of these evaluations justifies the methodological rigor, for example the use of specific time sampling methods, diary tools such as the Experience Sampling Method (ESM), also termed, Ecological Momentary Assessment (EMA), and the Diary Reconstruction Method (DRM), which accurately evaluates an individual's experience 'online' over time, also in particular activities and situations. These tools could be veritable information sources on how people use their time and the benefits or otherwise, they derived in so doing, among others, which could help in policy debates and formulation. With the potential pervasive ramifications of well-being and happiness, we no doubt need to continue on refining our approaches to evaluation them with a view to utilizing the findings in policy development and implementation. Nonetheless, that there is an increasing tendency toward greater emphasis on these measures worldwide underscores the greater role that they would likely play in future policy matters in not just the health but also other domains. Should we therefore not increasingly focus on these apparently benign issues more before they transform into 'wolves' literally devouring our health systems and should we not do so now? Is it not therefore that the increasing paradigmatic shift in the healthcare delivery with the patient at the center of activities is movement in the appropriate direction? Should we not therefore institute the necessary mechanisms to facilitate its actualization, for example, acknowledging the significant role that healthcare information and communication technologies would play in so doing, and actually taking measures to promote the widespread adoption and use of these technologies? The veneer of innocence that ignorance of the benefits of healthcare information and communication technologies confers belies the gravity of the consequences of its perpetuation, the need for us to be more proactive about achieving the dual healthcare delivery objectives therefore not just urgent, but imperative. After all what would we do with the information emanating from the surveys mentioned above, if not belatedly then, to fix problems that needed not arise in the first place. The point here is that in seeking solutions to healthcare delivery problems, we often miss the easiest yet potentially deadliest issues, and hence their solutions, which in fact, might partly at least explain why the problems with our health systems persist. The irony of it all is that the solutions to such problems are often much cheaper than those they require later, complicated, and deadly, the increased costs in hospitalization rates and stays, the expensive prescription medications needed to treat them, and costs of their long term treatment for examples, all avoidable preventing them. Yet, it seems not to be the case that many health systems are willing to invest resources in for examples the healthcare ICT that could be the engine driving a variety of initiatives, for examples, health education, health promotion, and disease prevention, capable of preventing many of the chronic diseases, whose course then manifest in many cases as described above. Does the seeming innocence of the antecedents of these conditions, then succeed in fooling us, for example in the 'nothing wrong' attitude in taking another of that 'unhealthy' meal? Perhaps we need a change in orientation regarding the sort of health information we feed the public, in not just form, but more significantly in content. May be we need to do something else to drive the point harder home regarding the need for the healthcare consumer as we noted earlier to recognize the responsibilities that come with the ever increasing rights that they would have regarding health matters. These are after all rights tied to those of everyone else, and whose recognition, again which we need to ensure somehow, of the stakes we all have in ensuring society's overall well-being and happiness, is not just as crucial, but would likely impel the recognition similarly, by the individual healthcare consumer. In other words, the information asymmetry that we mentioned above, which rectifying the widespread adoption and use of healthcare ICT would certainly help facilitate, is the core issue in the realization of our quest to achieve the dual healthcare delivery objectives. The elementary, secondary, and other stages involved in the exercise, that eventually lead to ensuring happiness, and well-being, at the individual and societal levels would depend not just on the availability of relevant information, but also on what people do with it. No doubt we have some way to go in achieving both, it is suspect how much emphasis we have thus far placed on the latter component of this exercise, which perhaps explains why it is not that people do not know the health risks of an unhealthy lifestyle is why they persist in it. Thus, our efforts need in addition to providing information, also doing so in ways, perhaps utilizing contextualized healthcare ICT that would make the information more effective in convincing individuals to embrace healthier lifestyles. These issues underline the importance of the life assessment surveys mentioned earlier, which could reveal issues that addressing would help some make the switch to healthy living. It is certainly worth the while, even necessary to recognize the significance of these issues and to explore ways to addressing them. Failed efforts in areas wherein such failures might be difficult to explain to generations to come that might blight the future of healthcare delivery must trouble many. This is more so considering the amount of information for example that we have on the health risks of cigarettes, while we still end up spending hundreds of millions of dollars treating smoking-related diseases, these upcoming generations likely to inherit some of the bill. Should we not then be more determined to prevent this happening, even if only from an ethico-moral perspective, and would it therefore be wrong to consider the options that we have in so doing, which would in the final analysis, unlikely suit everyone, and should this be sufficient reason not to explore those options, or should it not? Each health jurisdiction would have to consider these options primarily in the context of the overall national healthcare delivery goals, for example, stipulated in the Canada Health Act, an embodiment of the certain fundamental principles held dear by Canadians regarding health and healthcare delivery.

Thus, health jurisdictions, faced with pressures from many directions, legal, budgetary, socio-political, and from the expectations of the citizenry of the health services, would increasingly have to make complex decisions on healthcare delivery. However, such decisions would increasingly reflect evident considerations of the health/macroeconomic dyadic. In other words, the survival of health systems would depend ever more on the healthcare consumer, whose operations in the healthcare delivery scheme would be crucial to the country's macroeconomic health. Regardless of the funding system of health services therefore, every health system would have to 'embed' in its strategic thinking, what it has to do to ensure the delivery of affordable, accessible, safe, and qualitative health services to the healthcare consumer, cost-effectively, and efficiently. Even if the healthcare consumer did not know the full reasons for receiving so much attention, essentially, one the moral obligation to alleviate the pain and suffering of the healthcare consumer, and two, which in certain circuitous ways ties with the first, to ensure that the country's economy does not collapse, we must persevere in achieving the DHDO. Whereas the achievement of the DHDO would be easier were every healthcare stakeholder to have this information, as it would then raise the perceived and indeed the actual stake in the efforts to achieve the DHDO. The same argument would apply to regimes worldwide, in particular in many developing countries, oblivious to the depreciation in the quality of life that would pervade their countries, including themselves and their families, not adhering to principles that would ensure not just that their countries survive but also thrive. An extension of these principles explains why such regimes must crumble in the end, in an implosion, which no one but themselves would be able to stop. The problem is the delay in reversing such waning processes that not doing so earlier causes, which as we noted with the course of chronic diseases above, the longer the delay, the more expensive the reversal, if at all possible, and of course the longer it is. It is possible that heeding the advice Sachs gave mentioned earlier as soon as possible would help many of these low and middle-income countries redirect the health of their peoples and their economies, but as we have argued thus far, even industrialized countries need to continue to invest in the health sector. Both developed and developing economies also need to promote the use of healthcare information and communication technologies in the delivery of health services, taking the infrastructure and institutions in existence, into consideration, the emphasis on deployment also dependent on other health and non-health related variables, for examples, disease pattern and prevalence. Indeed, as with most other aspects of contemporary existence these two worlds would ultimately need each other in making their efforts at achieving the DHDO succeed. It is the combination of the aggregate of the will to survive in both worlds that would ultimately for example significantly contribute to the implosion mentioned earlier regarding regimes that ignore the fundamental aspirations of the majority to survive, an exercise that a variety of factors could accelerate or slow down, inherent in such regimes, and external to them. This is why the alliances countries form, are crucially dependent on their interests, meaning specifically, that to survive, rooted at an individual level. These alliances, specific and general, among other factors therefore determine the attention given to their partners in a variety of domains, including health. The point in reiterating these perhaps obvious facts is that in the end, each country and health jurisdiction would have to face its healthcare delivery challenges itself, in the main, and by extension, its economic survival. This further underscores the urgency with which all countries should take Sachs' advice. The interesting thing about so doing is the benefits accruable from just initial investments in health in certain instances, geared in the appropriate direction, for example, in implementing healthcare ICT, which could help immensely in the achievement of the DHDO. In a world in which the most fundamental right we have, which is to life, is increasingly precarious and its realization simultaneously complex, making its conceptualization more in virtual than in concrete terms, holding tight to the proverbial last straw, in this instance wellness and health, becomes increasingly pragmatic yet exigent. Focusing on improving the health, happiness, and well-being of Canadians therefore should be top priority. It is by so doing that we could confidently expect not just the individual to claim the right to life met, but also society as a whole, a necessary requirement from which the claim of meeting other rights would be possible, and the progress of society, and indeed, of the country, guaranteed. The position of researchers on the concept of maximizing collective happiness as a social welfare function is contentious, some researchers arguing that such a stance ignores evidence from political economics and research on happiness[6]. Frey and Stutzer (2006)[6] insisted that rather we should aim to improve the processes via which individuals could express their choices, to enable them develop and promote their concept of the good life, both individually and as a group. The point in fact is that it is no longer tenable that a person's well-being is simply a private experience, which we would find difficult to measure directly hence, as economists would customarily argue, we should focus on indirect measures such as expressed behavior. This is because research evidence abounds for the evaluation of the so-called 'subjective' experienced utility or well-being[7], its intuitive correlation with variables such as positive emotion, optimism, sociability, and reduced suicide risk also backed by research evidence[8,9], including from functional magnetic resonance imaging (fMRI), with brain activities more on the left than right prefrontal cortex in happy persons[10,11]. There is no doubt therefore that, as all other countries, we in Canada, ought to start to pay close attention to the happiness of Canadians, as an additional measure of the country's 'wealth' besides traditional measures such as the Gross National Product (GNP), among others. In fact, the GNP would decline in tandem with happiness hence we should measure the latter from time to time across the country, to ensure its status, and potential effect, positive or negative on the economy, with a view to fostering the former, and averting the latter. Indeed, since even so-called rational persons could be unreasonable in their actions, despite knowledge of the risks involved in those actions, revealed choices could not be entirely valid, except given full rationality, and as experts would contend, in applied cost benefit analysis, the technique of the choice made, contingent valuation in particular, key[6]. The choices we make are therefore not necessarily correct choices hence more prospects might not necessarily mean increased utility, which puts classical utilitarianism and its extensions in economics, the maximization of evaluated happiness as a surrogate for social welfare in jeopardy[11,12]. The use of collective happiness or national well-being, subjective well-being the starting point, as such a substitute, and to shepherd policy formulation are gaining increasing currency as this circumvents some of the criticisms of the former approach[13], enabling us to focus on individual subjective happiness. Indeed, research indicates that life satisfaction measures or other measures of 'happiness' for example quality of life (QOL), and well-being, could be and complement other measures of national income, and are invaluable measures of individual welfare. However, despite the growing body of knowledge on the value of aggregating social welfare as a social function measure, serious objections exist among experts on this issue, not least regarding potential problems interpersonal comparisons of happiness, although research evidence increasingly indicate the possibility of such comparison of utility[6]. New research also counters other objections, for example regarding the potential for cardinal and not just only ordinal measurement of utility, distortions due to political predilection for personal, ideological, and special interests, and individuals' distortions of the extent of happiness to sway government policy, among others. Despite these objections, these new researches essentially indicate the potential existence of many social welfare functions, that subjective well-being are valid indicators of individual welfare, more valuable and useful in conjunction with the maximization of GNP and other standard economic variables, albeit fully cognizant of the potential significance of other aspects of an individual that contribute to health. In other words, we need to ensure that we are not just considering individual happiness, but all other aspects that not only result in it, but that are crucial for the buoyancy of an individual's overall health, lacking which that individual would unlikely be happy in any case. We also need to appreciate the significance of the interrelatedness of individuals, and the overall national 'happiness,' or health in general, and by extension, economic growth and development. Canada therefore needs to strengthen current institutions and establish new ones that would ensure that such distortions of aggregate well-being as mentioned above do not occur, which only by so ensuring could we guarantee individual choice fulfillment, and that our happiness measures truly reflect the country's health and wealth being, including of its economy. Thus indeed, rather than aim for progressive monolithic improvement, we should establish from our surveys of life satisfaction, and indeed, all our measures of happiness, valuable pointers to a deeper appreciation of individual happiness, via a continuous dialogue among all individual and political stakeholders. This should be within the context of an evolving socio-political process, and by extension policy that these pointers, for examples the effects of time availability and usage on individual well-being, societal norms on the adolescent female, family size on work ethics, and direct to consumer advertising (DTC) on children, and the outcomes of the ongoing dialogue in essence, shape.

This approach emphasizes the focus of policy being on improving the mechanisms by which individuals make and meet the choices important to them in the realization of happiness, and in effect, the health, of both themselves as individuals, and as a group, and indeed, as a society and a country. This implies focus on the means by which we could enhance these processes or mechanisms, including for example, investing in the appropriate information and communication technologies, in the relevant areas, for example health, indeed, upfront, based on the results of our measures of happiness, subjected to in-depth analyses, predicated on the ongoing dialogue mentioned earlier. It would be necessary therefore, with regards health, for individuals to be able to express their preferences, make choices regarding their health matters, and indeed, in regard all matters that contribute directly or indirectly to their happiness. They should also be able to do so individually and as groups, the advancement of the nature and quality of the mechanisms involved in so doing, a crucial aspect of the accomplishment of the individual and collective happiness of Canadians. We should therefore have more than such bodies as Health Council of Canada, an independent council informing Canadians on health care matters simultaneously promoting accountability and transparency established in 2003, with the acceptance by the Prime Minister and the Premiers of the recommendations of the Kirby Report (October 2002) and the Romanow Commission (November 2002). There should also be mechanisms via which as noted earlier, Canadians are able to express their preferences for healthcare delivery and related issues and in general to further their concept of the good life, as individuals, and as communities. It is important however that we create the enabling environment for this to happen, highlights the need for such bodies as the Health Council of Canada, but also that of others that could provide Canadians the necessary information that could make for more discerning and healthier choices. This is not just in the best interests of the individual Canadians, but also by extension, that of the country and underscores the need for us to pay attention to the underlying processes involved in these bidirectional information exchanges. This also underscores the need for process cycle analyses by health jurisdictions to determine the issues, including those emanating from our life satisfaction and other 'happiness' surveys conducted regularly, provincially, territorially, and nationally, and the outcomes of the bidirectional exchanges mentioned above, germane to improving on an ongoing basis, the efficiency and effectiveness of healthcare delivery and all health-related issues. These analyses, which would involve progressive decomposition and exposition of issues and their processes, would reveal the appropriate processes to modify, those to facilitate, or expunge, for examples, and the relevant information technologies to deploy in so doing. These analyses would entail the synthesis of information from the various sources mentioned above, for example, from research evidence and new medical knowledge in general, as inputs into the decomposition/exposition exercises, for example, recent research findings by scientists on the workings of the brain circuitry that inoculate against stress, the circuitry of resilience[14]. The research published in the December 20, 2006 issue of *The Journal of Neuroscience* found that experiencing control over a stressor immunizes a rat from developing a depression-like syndrome when in future faced with stressors it cannot control. The researchers found that control activated the brain's executive hub, the prefrontal cortex, but in addition modified it, setting in motion later even confronted with uncontrollable stressors, the activation switching off mood-modulating cells in the brainstem's alarm core, making uncontrollable stressors seem controllable, giving an illusion of control, creating resilience confronted with adversity. Researches such as these would help us understand better how the brain handles the experience of control to protect us against future adversity. With lack of control over stressors major aspects of mood and anxiety disorders, such understanding would also help us develop more effective treatment modalities for these disorders, for example those aimed at enhancing perceived control, or coping, or the cortex's control over the brainstem and other stress-responsive structures. Such efforts would no doubt help reduce the prevalence of these disorders, and increase the levels of happiness and well-being at individual, hence collective levels. Could we not in fact develop effective approaches to psychological approaches 'training' the frontal cortex in this regard, inculcating in individuals at an early age, the knowledge and skills required to 'immunize' against stressors, with at least the potential to minimize their more damaging effects? This example illustrates the multidimensional nature of the efforts required to enhance the individual and collective happiness of Canadians, and the importance of so doing for the welfare of all, and the economic growth and development crucial to sustaining that of the country's health/economy dyadic. What would be the benefits of investing substantially on medical research for example, if the information emanating from such researches does not reach healthcare providers, or the healthcare consumer, who both need the information, one to improve treatment options, for example, the other, to facilitate the understanding of issues relating to health and disease, hence rational decision making, for example. These activities by both no doubt have important implications not only for the happiness in fact of both, not to underestimate the health benefits to the doctor for example, of merely being able to help patients, whose health improved would likely enhance well-being, but also for their families, and friends, society, and the country. Similarly, what would be the need for our 'happiness' surveys and other methods/exercises in measuring happiness, if we did not utilize the results in the bidirectional exchanges mentioned earlier, or in formulating policies that would further enhance the happiness of Canadians, and in effect the country's economic prosperity? It is clear therefore, that we need to start to pay attention to some seemingly benign issues to which if we did not, however, we risk the emergence of their true potential not just to compromise the happiness of individuals, but also, by extension, that of the country, including its economy. In other words, health matters that might seem at first harmless, might, on scrutiny turn out to be malevolent. Happiness is an attribute we take for granted and do not generally link, at least not by many, immediately, to national economy, many unlikely to consider the need for them to be happy anything other than a personal matter, or at least not that their country's economy hinges on it. As part of the information exchange process mentioned earlier, part of what we should be doing is letting Canadians know how important it is for them to be happy, and what the collective happiness of Canadians means to the progress of the country, and the latter for our continuing enjoyment of the good life to which we are so accustomed. As also previously noted, ideological, personal, and special interests aside, all Canadians need to realize what it at stake were we to ignore these basic principles, that the downturn in the country's economy would significantly impair all facets of life and business, and alienate the electorate anyway, paving the way for the downfall of the government at the earliest convenience. This is an important aspect of the cardinality/ordinality argument of the potential of happiness as social welfare functions, and the comparability of personal notions of happiness as in the final analysis, happiness is manifest when an individual is alive, and life satisfaction, implies there is life. It matters little therefore, if at all, the path by which individuals achieve this fundamental goal of staying alive, as it is unlikely that it would involve exercises that would overall hinder another individual from so doing, since the fundamental biological mechanisms involved in staying alive are universal. This does not mean that one individual could not derive 'joy' from hurting another, which underscores the need for policy in the first place of the sort mentioned earlier that promotes via the mechanisms mentioned earlier and others, the pursuit of happiness that would enhance that of the individual, and that of the group, society, and country. Thus, we need to promote mechanisms that reinforce such cherished Canadian values as those enshrined in the Charter of Rights, starting with the right to life, and those in the Canada Health Act, which complement them with regard healthcare delivery. We also need, in the process, to promote a deeper understanding by Canadians, via the dialogue and exchanges mentioned earlier, among other measures, of the need for them to be healthy, hence happy, and not just individually, but also collectively. This would be key approaches to averting the negative aspects of the competitiveness that the right to life implies, including for example, the tendency by some to derive their happiness trampling on the rights of others to be equally happy, hence healthy, fostering that of collaboration, in a collective effort to ensure the survival, and progress of the country. These exercises would reduce if not eliminate the maneuverability by individuals and politicians alike of the happiness levels that constitute a major criticisms by classical welfare economic theorist of aggregate happiness being a valid indicator of social welfare.

Happiness as we have noted has macro-and micro-economic relevance. At the former level, its advantages over customary economic indicators of social welfare for example, the GNP, are considerable. Given the phenomena, economists call hedonic adaptation and the aspiration treadmill, the effects of life events changes on happiness being only temporary, and could potentially modify an individual's aspirations, respectively, again as earlier noted, we need to be wary of a monolithic social function approach to happiness. This would mean not predicating policy for example solely on the capacity or otherwise of an individual for adaptation, for example, but rather on a thorough appreciation of the effects on adaptation of the various processes involved in happiness, as the research on the 'circuitry of resilience' earlier mentioned shows, and ways by which we could enhance these processes. This example also underscores the need also mentioned earlier for the individual, and with reference to health being the progenitor of happiness, the healthcare consumer, being central. In other words, viewed from whichever perspective, the individual Canadian should feature most prominently in how we construct our political processes, the fundamental premise of which should be to ensure that the individual and collective interests of Canadians take precedence over any other consideration. The centrality of the individual recognizes the fulfillment of individual preferences as a key objective of policy formulation, which to arrive at as the ultimate outcomes, in synthesizing inputs from our happiness researches, grounded in the dialogue and exchange processes mentioned earlier, the resulting policies essentially ensure. It is not enough to pay lip service literally to the concept of the centrality of the individual if we were to achieve these objectives. We actually need to establish the institutions and other mechanisms that would ensure that we achieve what we set out to adopting this perspective of the central position of the individual Canadian, the personal preferences fulfillment in tandem with collective happiness crucial to the progress, albeit survival of Canada as a country. Our approach should emphasize the significance of individual happiness, and the need for research evidence of its indicators, but not on wholesale politico-bureaucratic intervention-fiat on outcome enhancement that directly measured, maximized aggregates of happiness dictate, but on an in-depth appreciation of the processes involved, to determine the appropriate ways to improve the latter, hence outcomes. That Canada is a developed country neither means that we cannot strengthen existing institutions and mechanisms to ensure we achieve these objectives, whereas in fact, given that change is a continuous process, the need for us to establish new ones would always arise, as no system is, at least in theory perfect. This tendency for systems to be inherently unstable is positive only were we to appreciate the need for the continued process improvement that the increasingly sophisticated aspirations and expectations of Canadians, regarding healthcare delivery for example, entail. In other words, we would then appreciate as even more urgent the need to establish the relevant mechanisms and institutions to ensure this perpetual process and in effect quality improvement. With regard health, this would lead us essentially to the quest to achieve the dual healthcare delivery objectives (DHDO), the ultimate goals in which process improvement in healthcare delivery would result. One of the first tasks of every health jurisdiction in the country therefore, would be accepting the fact that whatever they are doing now is imperfect, and that their healthcare jurisdiction could never be perfect. This is by no means an easy task for any leader, be it at the provincial, health region, hospital, or at any other level, however, this is only if that individual saw the acknowledgement of these facts as an indictment of their managerial acumen, and an acceptance of failure, but is far from being the case. It is necessary for such individuals to recognize that it is just a sort of clean slate upon which a new approach to strategic management would hinge. It aims to facilitate the emphasis of the health jurisdiction on the centrality of the healthcare consumer, an emphasis that would result in dramatic changes in both the conceptualization and delivery of health services. This newness whim did not spawn, but the equally dramatic changes in contemporary healthcare zeitgeist did. It is thus the case that every Canadian healthcare jurisdiction needs to embrace these developments and as quickly as possible as they would in the end were they to survive let alone thrive. Not doing so now though would not only mean taking longer to catch-up, but also having to face down the road economic losses due to current policies, which would be clear in the end were flawed. To be sure, these economic losses would encompass dimensions wider than the health jurisdiction in question, in both human and material terms. Besides the potential of major disruptions in health services organization in the jurisdiction, with possible the need to close down hospitals that have lost patronage, to more competitive jurisdictions, even within Medicare, and are no longer economically viable, and to merge others, there is the depletion of the 'happiness pool' and denting of the country's overall economy to contend with. This is not to mention the ethico-moral issues involved in depriving the individual Canadian the opportunity to meet his/her preferences in healthcare delivery, and of course thus jeopardizing his/her happiness, and overall health, essentially infringing on his/her right to life. Each health jurisdiction therefore needs after acknowledging the facts of the need for continuous quality evaluation and improvement, to embark on the means to so doing. This underlines the need for these health jurisdictions to create the enabling environment for the expression by individual Canadians and collectively, of their concepts of the good life, and their expectations of their health systems, which met, would contribute immensely to the achievement of happiness by the citizenry. As trivial as these issues might sound to some, they are the mimicry of a lamb. With health spending by Canada ever increasing, population aging increasingly a potential burden on health services utilization and costs, the country's workforce not increasing significantly, and immigration creating new healthcare delivery challenges, amongst others, ignoring these issues could unleash a health crisis the true extent of which would astonish many. Despite the projected slight increase in external markets in 2007, the country's domestic demand would decelerate moderately in the wake of its recent strong expansion, and inflation pressures billed to remain restricted, with falls in energy prices from recent peaks, wages not expected to increase appreciably[15]. Is it any surprise therefore that the Organization for Economic Cooperation and Development (OECD) counseled on the need for fiscal settings at all levels of government in the country to remain prudent and for the federal government to concentrate on reducing the debt burden before pressure due to population aging piles up? With a significant proportion of this pressure being on health services, does it not make intuitive sense for health jurisdictions to attempt to reduce health spending simultaneously improving the quality of healthcare delivery? Would it not in fact make sense however perceived for health jurisdictions to embrace the DHDO, which essentially enables the achievement of these twin goals? Finally, would be unreasonable for health jurisdictions to invest in the healthcare information and communication technologies crucial to the achievement of these dual healthcare delivery goals? The point here is that there are indications that health jurisdictions in Canada would have to embrace not just the idea of the DHDO, but the technologies that make the achievement of these goals possible[16]. To incorporate the indicators of happiness that would emerge from surveys into policy formulation would involve determining the most efficient and cost-effective ways to implement these policies, essentially, to enhance the processes involved in fulfilling the personal preferences of Canadians in meeting their happiness goals, hence by extension health goals. This overall would coincide with the collective health objectives of Canadians in the main hence promote the country's economic growth and productivity. It is unlikely therefore that there would any significant opposition to any policy aimed at facilitating disease prevention and health promotion initiatives, which derive from the dialogue and information exchange processes mentioned earlier. Thus, health jurisdictions would need to determine the most appropriate programs based on the specificities of their particular jurisdictions, within the context of overall national healthcare delivery goals as embodied in the Canada Health Act. They would also need to determine the relevant healthcare ICT to deploy in their actualization, within the framework of the national health information network that Canada Health Infoway oversees, for example. The need for collaboration at national, provincial and territorial levels for example, obvious in the efforts at the local levels in implementing the relevant healthcare ICT yielding better results, in the overall national framework, which is the ultimate goal as our discussion thus far emphasizes. It is obvious in that to a major extent the integration of the national and local efforts at implementing these technologies facilitates the achievement of this ultimate goal, and the lack of it, slows down progress in the achievement of the DHDO, at all levels. Determining the most appropriate programs for any jurisdiction is a major exercise, which itself predicates on embracing another important concept that of process cycle analysis. Thus, the outcomes of the determinants of happiness that emerges from the various happiness estimation that health jurisdictions would conduct, would constitute the inputs for the dialogue, and information exchanges mentioned earlier, and for the process cycle analyses required to facilitate policy formulation and implementation. These exercise would enable the health jurisdiction determine which processes to modify, and which healthcare information and communication technologies for example, to deploy in so doing.

The connection between individual happiness and health in general, and Canada's overall economic growth and development is certain, as is the need for Canadians to know this in the new Canada. Indeed, a crucial aspect of the application of insights from happiness research, more of which we would have to engage in, is the elimination of information asymmetry, enabling information flow across multiple domains, including to the individual Canadian. This would facilitate the appreciation by this person, of the true meaning of happiness or put differently the good life, and its importance to the achievement of the most cherished right of all, that to life, on the one hand. It would also foster the appreciation of the significance of the rights of other Canadians to achieve that right, and of its achievement to the survival, economic growth, and sustainable development of the country. Here again, we see the crucial role that these technologies could play in eliminating information asymmetry. The need for the

Canadian health system to embrace these technologies is not just urgent, but imperative. Not that these technologies are absent within the health system, but that we could use them even more in several aspects of the healthcare delivery enterprise. Furthermore, integrating these technologies at all levels of healthcare delivery and among different healthcare stakeholders is a requirement for the realization of their full potential in helping us achieve the dual healthcare delivery objectives (DHDO.) Finally, it seems quite obvious the potential for wastage of scarce resources that not integrating these disparate and essentially stand-alone healthcare ICT currently in existence even within healthcare jurisdictions, means for Canada Health Infoway, for example, but also for health jurisdictions across the country. Canada Health Infoway whose goal is to have an interoperable EHR implemented across 50% of Canada (by population) by the end of 2009, has invested substantially in a variety of projects nationwide towards achieving this goal, as have health jurisdictions in the country. Yet, not integrating these systems means not achieving their full potential, including helping us achieve the dual healthcare delivery objectives, and it is important that we do. There is no doubt about the achievements of Medicare, but with health spending on the increase, 9.9% of GDP in Canada in 2004 and increasing, we should not expect a trouble-free health system down the road. Costs, which would likely increase due to ageing populations, among others, and increased demand on services with heightened expectations by seniors of the quality and outcomes health services, among other factors would be key challenges that the country's health system would confront in the years ahead. As we have attempted to show in this discussion, hard economics variables, in this instance measures such as the number of hospital beds per 1000 patients, would be increasingly less important to the healthcare consumer, as performance measures of their health system and indeed of policy measures as would outcome measures. Predicated on the increasingly complex expectations of the ever more suave healthcare consumer, the increasing significance of outcome measures underscores the points we have made about that of happiness, and the increasing centrality of the healthcare consumers, all of which would have a significant influence on healthcare delivery in Canada in the future. This is why we cannot afford to ignore these emerging developments, and not prepare our health system for the challenges ahead. These issues have close links with some of the most cherished values of Canada, for example, the right to life, which is the fundamental reason we cannot but take the necessary measures that would enable the achievement of this right by all Canadians. Such measures as improving the quality of healthcare delivery, at the same time reducing health spending would no doubt help in achieving this objective, which would ensure that the individual Canadian meets his/her preferences. They would also guarantee that all Canadians do, and in so doing, create the enabling environment for the country's economy to thrive, an interest in which we all share. Considering the intense competitiveness on the global markets, every Canadian has the duty to contribute toward, and no matter how little, the success of the country in its efforts to enable us continue to enjoy the enviable standards of living that we currently do. It is the responsibility of all of us and of government to ensure that we all know this. In other words, the healthcare consumer not only derives benefits from the health system, he/she has responsibilities to the health system too. One such duty is not to overuse the services and incur unnecessary costs on frivolous procedures and treatments that they really do not need. Thus, as our health system obviates the need for worries about moral hazard and adverse selection, because Medicare is in the main free, over-burdening the system would compromise the availability of resources we need to maintain the standards of care that we currently enjoy and even improve upon them. There are of course a number of other issues that we need to address regarding our health system, the overall goal, regardless that of the achievement of the dual healthcare delivery objectives, which goals, not only relate to ensuring best outcomes and happiness for the healthcare consumer, but also the achievement of the our country's growth and economic development. It is the pursuit of these goals that would likely be the major preoccupations of healthcare delivery in Canada in the years ahead, and it is likely that we will given the country's track record of being able to manage its resources admirably, while still loyal to commitments on the ideals of the Canadian peoples over the years.

References

1. Frey, Bruno S. and Schneider, F. (1978). "An Empirical Study of Politico-Economic Interaction in the US", Review of Economics and Statistics, 60(2), 174-183.

2. Di Tella, R., MacCulloch, R., Oswald, J., The macroeconomics of happiness. OECD 2001

3. Kahneman, Daniel, and Richard Thaler (1991). "Economic Analysis and the Psychology of Utility: Applications to Compensation Policy", American Economic Review, 81(2), 341-6.

4. Kahneman, Daniel, Wakker, Peter and Rakesh Sarin, (1997). "Back to Bentham? Explorations of Experienced Utility", Quarterly Journal of Economics, 112, 375-406.

5. Available at: http://www.accessmylibrary.com/coms2/summary_0286-66365_ITM Accessed on December 17, 2006

6. Frey, B.S., Stutzer, A., Should We Maximize National Happiness? Institute for Empirical Research in Economics, University of Zurich, Working Paper Series ISSN 1424-0459, Working Paper No. 306, October 2006

7. Kahneman, D., Krueger, A.B., (2006) Developments in the Measurement of Subjective Well-Being. *Journal of Economic Perspectives* 20(1): 3-24.

8. Frey, B.S., Stutzer, A., (2002b). What Can Economists Learn from Happiness Research? *Journal of Economic Literature* 40(2): 402-35.

9. Honkanen., K, Honkanen, H.R., Viinamaki, H., Heikkila, K., et. al. (2001). Life Satisfaction and Suicide: A 20-Year Follow-up Study. *American Journal of Psychiatry* 158(3): 433-439.

10. Zak, Paul J. (2004). Neuroeconomics. *Philosophical Transactions of the Royal Society of London Series B-Biological Sciences* 359(1451): 1737-1748.

11. Pugno, Maurizio (2004). Rationality and Affective Motivations: New Ideas from Neurobiology and Psychiatry for Economic Theory? Discussion Paper No. 1, Department of Economics, University of Trento

12. Tinbergen, Jan (1956). *Economic Policy: Principles and Design*. Amsterdam: North Holland.

13. Layard, Richard (2005). *Happiness: Lessons from a New Science*. New York: Penguin.

14. Available at: http://www.nimh.nih.gov/press/stress-resilience.cfm
Accessed on December 23, 2006

15. Available at: http://www.oecd.org/document/52/0,2340,en_2649_201185_19726196_1_1_1_1,00.html Accessed on December 23, 2006

16. Available at: http://www.healthcareitnews.com/story.cms?id=3653
Accessed on December 23, 2006

The Wait Times Issue

Preventable adverse events, medical errors resulting in harm to a patient should not occur, but they do. The U.S., Institute of Medicine (IOM) report, 'To Err is Human: Building A Safer Health System,' released on November 01, 1999, showed that at least 44,000 people, possibly up to 98,000 people, die in hospitals every year due to preventable medical errors[1]. The report recommended measures to reduce medical errors and improve patient safety stressing the existence of the expertise to implement them, setting a minimum target of 50% reduction in medical errors in five years, in achieving which, emphasizing the need for balance between regulatory and market forces, and between professionals and organizations. Another IOM report, released in 2001 'Crossing the Quality Chasm: A new health System for the 21st century,' lamented the frequent harm that healthcare in the U.S., does to patients and its failure to meet its full potential, the lag not a gap, but a chasm[2], to close which it stressed the need for radical health system and policy transformations. Yet, medical errors, which IOM defines as the failure of a planned action to be completed as intended or the use of a wrong plan to achieve an aim, persists, and are of different types, for examples, adverse drug events (ADEs), wrong-site surgeries, incorrect transfusions, falls, surgical injuries , burns, suicides, mistaken patient identities, restraint-related injuries, and pressure sores, among others[3]. At the behest of the Senate Finance Committee, the U.S. Congress via the Medicare Modernization Act of 2003 (Section 107(c)), mandated that Centers for Medicare and Medicaid Services sponsor a study by the IOM to study the prevalence and costs of medication errors and devise a national agenda for reducing them, among other objectives. The report found that medication errors are not just common, occurring in hospitals, at every step of the medication process, from procuring the drug, to prescribing, dispensing, and administering it, even evaluating its impact, in particular during prescribing and administering, but costly to the country. An ADE due to an error is technically, preventable, and with annual estimates by various studies of preventable, ADEs according to this report in hospitals between 380,000 and 450,000, in long-term care (LTC) facilities, 800,000, and among outpatient Medicare patients, 530,000, some, for examples the hospital figures, even deemed underestimates, the problem is enormous. Indeed, the report estimated considering these numbers, which it also noted omitted errors of omission, not prescribing medication where it should, at least 1.5 million preventable ADEs occur yearly in the country, this estimate it considered likely an underestimate, and recommended an inclusive approach to reducing the prevalence of these errors necessitating pervasive system changes involving all healthcare stakeholders. Medication errors are also costly, in human and material terms, each preventable ADEs in a hospital, according to one study, increasing the cost of hospital stay about $8,750 (in 2006 dollars) more expensive. Thus, if there were 400,000 of such errors annually, costs would be $3.5 billion in just this group, estimates for treat medication errors in another, Medicare enrollees aged 65 years and older, $887 million annually[2]. Again, the report observed that these might be underestimates, as the medication errors examined were selective, as were the costs, for example, regarding the latter, excluding lost earnings and recompense for pain and suffering. Yet, many of these errors are preventable. Preventable medical errors are not peculiar to the U.S. They are also common in Canada, for example[4], according to the 2004 annual report by the Canadian Institute for Health Information (CIHI), 'Health Care in Canada 2004', which also noted significant regional/territorial differences in the performance of the country's health system. The report found that nearly 25% (1 in every 4 Canadians) (5.2 million people) indicated that they or a family member experienced a preventable, adverse event in 2003, including given wrong medication type/dose, or foreign objects left in the post-surgery, medical errors in Canada resulting in 1.1 million extra hospital days, with significant costs implications. Many of these errors are also preventable, and since a number of tested strategies and techniques exist for reducing medical errors, for example simply marking an ankle with a pen to make certain the surgeon did not operate on the wrong one, or implementing electronic prescribing, that these error still occur is no doubt unacceptable. So is therefore any delay in rectifying the problem, although we need first to know its causes, some of which we already know, but others, not so well, at least not all of their ramifications for healthcare delivery. Perhaps in the latter group would fall the findings of a recent study funded by the U.S. Department of Health & Human Service's (HHS) Agency for Healthcare Research and Quality (AHRQ) and the Centers for Disease Control and Prevention's National Institute for Occupational Safety and Health, and published on December 12, 2006 in the online journal *PLoS Medicine* [5]. According to this study, first-year trainee-doctors in the U.S. reported that working five extra-long shifts, of 24 hours or more at a time not resting, per month resulted in a 300% increase in the likelihood of a fatigue-related preventable adverse event that played a part in a patient's death. The study, which underlines findings in earlier similar studies and the increasing interests in patient safety and that of their doctors for that matter has potential major implications for resource development, allocation, and utilization, in health services delivery. With sleep-deprived interns that work 24-hour shifts likelier to make many more serious medical errors while working in intensive care units (ICUs) and crash their cars more frequently than those doctors working for just 16 consecutive hours, the implications for the training of interns would be quite profound. This is more so considering ongoing concerns in the U.S. that most interns work past the limits of a 2003 national standard that the Accreditation Council for Graduate Medical Education implemented and that they are likelier to injure themselves per chance, with a needle/other sharp instrument working in a hospital for over 20 consecutive hours, or working at night[5]. That the sample size in the study is sufficiently large to show that preventable adverse events rates spiral when interns work shifts of 24 hours or more underscores the multiple origins and dimensions of safety. It highlights the need in addressing this issue to consider, among others, the perspective of both the patient and the doctor, and the relationship of safety to such issues as hospital wait times, seemingly pervasive in many health systems, for which, limitations of professional work force, no doubt, at least in part, accounts. Thus, it might be that efforts to solve the problem with extended wait times to see healthcare providers, whose ethico-moral implications are profound besides its potential to increase the burden of disease, its costs, hence health spending, and at a fundamental philosophical level, to infringe on the rights of individuals, need to be more robust. Would it not be necessary for example, within the context of our desire to redress the perennial mal-distribution of doctors for example, to consider findings in the above study? Should we not for examples consider the findings indicating that interns were thrice likelier to report at least one fatigue-related preventable adverse event during months that they worked between one and four extended-duration shifts, seven times more so in those months they worked over five extended-duration shifts? What implications do the findings in the latter instance that these doctors were also likelier to fall asleep during lectures, rounds, and clinical activities, including surgery, for the quality of the knowledge and skills they acquired in training, and for the likelihood of their making even mistakes in their practice? There is no doubt about the potential adverse consequences of these issues for the quality of learning by doctors and that of patient care, with many doctors falling asleep driving home, and some doctors having died as a result, are we not also depleting the already inadequate pool of doctors, not addressing these issues? It is an open secret that interns routinely work extended shifts in teaching and other hospitals in many countries, including developed countries. Indeed, guidelines for graduate medical education in the U.S., for example, still allow up to nine 'marathon [30-hour long] shifts' per month, although there is a cap on the total number of hours worked, by the Accreditation Council on Graduate Medical Education (ACGME) since 1 July 2003, 80 hours a week. Interestingly, ACGME also stipulated that shifts should not last more than 24 hours, and residents would have a day off in seven and a 10-hour break between being on call and working a shift[6]. However, the reason for the 'marathon' is evident considering the Council's statement that 'Residents may remain on duty for up to 6 additional hours to participate in didactic activities, transfer care of patients, conduct outpatient clinics, and maintain continuity of medical and surgical care,' since virtually every U.S. medical resident could be held longer to perform these activities. Should part of our efforts to address the 'wait times' issue therefore not involve eliminating such loopholes, besides enforcing somehow the guidelines of such bodies in other countries, such as Canada? That the long shifts worked by interns, or any doctor for that matter, compromise the safety of both patients and doctors, and could, the quality overall of health delivery, with its implications, for increased morbidity and mortality, and eventually, health spending, with potential adverse consequences for the economy is not in doubt. What is in doubt is how much we attention we are paying to this vis-à-vis the wait times issue, and by extension to both, regarding our obligation to provide qualitative health services cost-effectively and efficiently?

Attributing health services provision to obligatory categories could seem inane to some, to clarify the justification for which assertion though, hardly stretches reason, considering the tendency to life than to death, in most of us. This tendency then implies that we in the main engage in activities that result in the former than in the latter or in which on aggregate result in the latter at least by default, given our proclivity sometimes for a seeming lack of reason, even then the preference of most for the former unsullied. Life-sustaining activities essentially include those communal, and complement and facilitate those singular aimed to achieve an individual's objective to live, which in turn, similarly fosters that of the community so to do, in a perpetual symbiotic dyadic. The evolutionary advantage of this deceptively simple process is evident all around us, competition an integral aspect of collaboration, the latter a more potent ingredient of survival, in competition, in particular in our times of milieus global, and ingeniously oftentimes described as 'hypercompetitive.' It is therefore exigent, and indeed, imperative for health services provision to all to feature high on the list of obligatory enterprises crucial for the achievement of the survival motive of the individual, in keeping with its coalescence with that of the community, so to do. The question then is moot that we might be compromising the abilities of both to survive doing otherwise. It is therefore important that we consider all the potential issues involved in the achievement of this objective of health services provision to all, including, perhaps most critically, the mechanisms involved therein, and their maneuverability in the context of the relevant issues at play in a particular health jurisdiction, in the actualization of the healthcare delivery enterprise. It is by focusing on these mechanisms for example that we could hope to solve the problem of wait times in our health jurisdiction. What we are advocating therefore is a new mindset regarding this problem that would enable us address in a systematic manner, the variety of issues, some of them directly, others remotely connected to yet critical in solving it. A key conclusion of the 1999 IOM report referred to earlier for example is that most medical errors do not result from the carelessness of an individual or a particular group, but from defective systems, processes, and conditions that result in individuals blundering or failing to avert them. Imagine the potential danger in a patient able to access and drink large quantities of say mouthwash, which would have a lot of alcohol in it, the patient being on medications whose interaction with alcohol could be life threatening. It is therefore important that we recognize the need to design our health system at all levels with safety sharply in focus, with regard the example given above, to keep the mouthwash securely locked up and inaccessible to patients, who only receive from staff the amount needed and when. In other words, a cardinal goal of this design is to make it more difficult and easier to engage in inappropriate and appropriate acts, respectively. Rather than apportioning blame on an individual when something goes awry, which is not to eschew vigilance or accepting responsibility, we should focus on identifying where in the system the problem is and devise the appropriate solution to fixing it, as we would this way likelier prevent a repeat of the error. Non-system errors could be sabotage, or related to personality flaws or illnesses, for example, visual problems, are easier to identify, and dealt with accordingly, offering the needed help to the individual, or taking other necessary measures to prevent the errors made happening again. The significant differences across Canada in some health performance indicators in the CIHI report mentioned earlier, for example, are grounds for a thorough system re-evaluation in these health jurisdictions. According to that report, in Nova Scotia, 24.2% of patients who had a stroke expired in hospital within 30 days, the rate in Alberta, 15.5%. Do these figures reveal differences in the quality of care, wait times, prescription practices, patient safety, or even flawed diagnostic workup? The answers to these questions would best emerge in the course of a thorough process cycle analyses, which by decomposing and exposing the constituent processes and issues involved in the management of these patients in both health jurisdictions, would no doubt reveal where problem areas are, and what to do to fix these problems. Thus, another critical approach to solving the 'wait times' problem is to embrace the use of data and information collated from relevant sources as input in an ongoing decomposition/exposition exercise, process cycle analyses, which would reveal the interplay of the various dimensions of the issue, hence the potential solutions to them. In addition, it would enable putting to test, via an evaluative analytical process, the value of these solutions in addressing and solving the problem. In other words, the 'wait times' issue is not static. The issues and processes that clog the healthcare delivery wheel literally are paradoxically motorized, changing dynamics, the mechanics of which we need to know and be able to tinker. This places the approach to solving the wait times issue in purely contextual domains within broad policy guidelines, predicated in Canada, for example, on the principles enshrined in the Canada Health Act. The dynamic nature of these issues and processes, which is not surprising considering what some would consider the frenetic pace of progress in medical knowledge, for example, means that any measures aimed at solving the wait times problem would soon become obsolete not based in the first place on this scalable premise. Thus, every such effort must operate in tandem with the evolution of the health system of the jurisdiction in question, recognizing the fact that we could mandate as a national guideline, more specifically than does Canada, for example, the dictates of the core values of Canadians manifest in the Canada Health Act. Thus, besides the need for healthcare to be universal and accessible among others, the question arises whether to stipulate minimum acceptable wait times for specific or general. Alternatively, we might want to establish guidelines on wait times that would involve considerations of crucial local issues, such as the availability and distribution of healthcare professionals, the nature and severity of the illness, and the expertise required, and ICT usage, among others. Considering the aforementioned, it would no doubt be unrealistic to stipulate an all-inclusive wait time, as in theory, this might mean for some provinces or territories, outsourcing certain services, which in itself is not necessarily a bad thing, but which is best an integral strategic intent of that health jurisdiction, rather than being exigent upon imposed pressure. This issue highlights the difficulty in using aggregate measures of for example life satisfaction as a social welfare function, not least because of the difficulty of comparability of individual happiness, and regarding it, that of resolving the cardinality/ordinality conundrum of contemporary micro-economic welfare theory. Even if we based the parameters on the least onerous for every province or territory, we risk the sort of socio-political distortions that some might consider charlatanic. Yet, it is only intuitive not to expect every health jurisdiction to have the wherewithal, labor, and technology in particular, to meet the minimal requirements for waiting to see a cardiologist if one had angina pectoris, for example. Whereas, not only would the scientific, evidence-based guidelines serve benchmark purposes, the trail attaining it would be evident even to the lay what efforts the health jurisdiction is making or has made being adequate or otherwise. Such transparency of process improvement and its continuous evaluation toward the achievement of the benchmarks is precisely the sort of bidirectional ongoing healthcare consumer/provider dialogue conducted in keeping with democratic principles that would result in the appropriate solution to the 'wait times' problem in the end. Thus, it is unlikely that healthcare consumers in a particular healthcare jurisdiction that has only two family doctors would expect that just because Ottawa says no one should wait for more than two days to see the doctor, then everything would change and they would see their family doctors within that period, rather than the customary three. Whereas these healthcare consumers would be likelier more attuned to understanding the recruitment and retention efforts of their health jurisdiction, and be more willing to utilize the new virtual consultation technologies implemented to reduce wait times in the meantime, for example, being involved via ongoing dialogues in the efforts of the health jurisdiction. The point here is that we need to adopt a more flexible approach to solving the 'wait times' problem, one rooted in a clear-eyed appreciation of the many issues involved and their peculiarities to health jurisdictions that make fiat-like pronouncements even based on research evidence of the treatment of particular disorders not necessarily realistic in achieving 'wait times' reductions. As the example of the interns mentioned above shows, what if we actually caused more problems than we had making interns, surgeons, or any doctor work longer hours because we want to reduce 'wait times,' the very healthcare consumers we are trying to satisfy ending up dissatisfied, even suing us, for whatever reason? Should we rather not be ferreting, even if cryptic, systems issues obstructing the smooth operations of our health systems, adopting a flexible, multidimensional approach to solving the 'wait times' problem? Indeed, it is only in this regard that adopting a monolithic aggregate approach to addressing the issue would work, as the enunciates general principles, for example the deployment of process cycle analyses in decomposing and exposing systems issues for further decomposition/exposition exercises along a continuum of quality improvement and evaluation predicated on the inevitability of change, are essentially universal.

There is thus need for commonalities regarding wait-list management, including for example, and most importantly, what terminologies such as wait-times or 'excessive delays' for examples mean to all. In October 2005, the Canadian Institute for Health Information (CIHI) held a national conference on such issues although as noted earlier, the mobile and contextual nature of the key issues regarding wait times suggest that such measures be ongoing. It might be okay for example to recommend waiting no longer than a certain time period for a particular health condition or diagnostic procedure now but not so in another year or two due to the mergence of new knowledge or technologies, or evidence-based, management guidelines. One cannot gainsay the point about the futility in establishing rigid across-board 'wait times' limits independent of the outcomes of ongoing healthcare consumer/provider information exchange and dialogue within established democratic institutions and processes. Would it be necessary for patients to wait for surgery for a procedure for example, they know other treatment modalities would help overcome, or would the need for some complex cardiac procedure arise were individuals, not oblivious efforts they could make earlier to avert or attenuate known risk factors for the condition? Should we not examine and do something about individuals failing to show up for scheduled appointments, those missed appointments key contributors to extended, 'wait times'? Could we not attend to measures to reduce the moral hazard aspects of 'wait times' reduction, as part of our overall systems-focused approach to the problem? What role could the widespread implementation and use of healthcare information and communication technologies play in this regard, in particular rectifying information asymmetry, healthcare's atavistic relic? Do these questions not underscore the need for the sort of process cycle analyses mentioned earlier that would reveal the issues and sub-issues, processes and sub-processes necessary in adequately tackling this problem? There is no doubt that we would have to start to conceptualize the issues surrounding 'wait times' and their solutions more comprehensively in particular as the population ages, and the prevalence of chronic heart and musculo-skeletal conditions increases, both groups some of the chief reasons for complicated medical and surgical interventions, and major contributors to the 'wait times' problem. Our approaches to measuring, monitoring, and improving wait times would no doubt be within a certain framework to which all healthcare jurisdictions would subscribe. These would include for examples, general procedural principles, the deployment, and use of healthcare ICT for measuring, evaluating, and auditing general parameters, and the importation, testing and perhaps implementation with required modifications of tactical maneuvers, technical, managerial, and medical, proven effective in reducing wait times in other jurisdictions. These measures, however, would simply be a national framework, the particular modalities each jurisdiction uses essentially unique to that jurisdiction, determined via in-depth analytical processes cognizant of the peculiarities of that jurisdiction. As relative as it sounds, the approach advocated here is consistent with the operations of the foundations of the aggregate motion that result in actions characteristic of the individual desire, which in tandem with the communal, critically assures the right to life, that to health an intermediate process in the entire enterprise. In other words, our efforts as part of our process improvement efforts should also focus on reiterating the centrality of the healthcare consumer in the healthcare delivery scheme. Given the appropriate, current, and relevant information, the healthcare consumer so positioned would inevitably make the correct choices enough times not to disrupt the motion described above, more so, as not so doing is integral, and the healthcare consumer should also know, to the survival of the community, and indeed, of the country. With the increasing recognition of the use of psychological variables such as life satisfaction, quality of life, or simply happiness, as perhaps more heuristic measures of national welfare, and economic progress, than for example, traditional macro-economic variables such as gross national product (GNP), unemployment, and inflation figures the stakes in ensuring individual and communal health increasingly would be higher. This would make it much easier for us to exploit the fundamental interplay of factors involved in the actualization of healthcare delivery, which in turn would facilitate identifying and implementing the solutions to the many problems hampering its effectiveness and efficiency, including the 'wait times' issue. The point then is that in seeking solutions to this issue, we should situate our efforts squarely within the individual Canadian's health universe. We cannot solve the 'wait times' problem without the active involvement of the healthcare consumer. We need input from healthcare delivery end-users regarding their expectations of the services we deliver, or propose. These inputs are crucial in our policy formulation on healthcare accessibility issues, including 'wait times.' It is unlikely for example that the healthcare consumer would expect to 'jump the queue in the emergency room (ER) to see the doctor, but also so that he or she would be amused, waiting two hours so to do. Such considerations, many evident in our life satisfaction surveys, and in the outcomes of the ongoing dialogues and information exchange among other sources, should constitute elements of the additional national framework, which provinces and territories would incorporate in their contextualized approaches to solving the peculiar problems that confront their health systems, including the 'wait times' issue. Adopting a flexible functional approach, rather a rigid structural one creates opportunities for exploring issues the magnitude of whose effects on healthcare was hitherto unknown, or unanticipated. The centrality of the healthcare consumer for example no doubt creates additional pressure on the health system to deliver efficient and cost-effective health services. This pressure, coupled with others, for examples, budgetary constraints, and population aging, could be sufficiently intense to threaten the very existence of health services, even hospitals and health jurisdictions. Thus, health jurisdictions need to deliver qualitative services on the one hand, but also to do so within strict budgetary limits, which latter, the consequences of an increasingly aging population, for examples, increased demand for and utilization of services could severely test. The onus is therefore on health jurisdictions to aim to achieve the dual healthcare delivery objectives (DHDO.) The consequences of the alternatives of increased taxes or devolution of healthcare coverage could be equally grave for the overall health of the citizenry to be precise. Indeed, because the pressures of the motion described above toward health would hardly permit either, this onus becomes mandatory. In other words, the decline in the discretionary spending power that increased taxation to fund healthcare would engender would itself ultimately result in the decline in QOL that could compromise health, besides making less resources available for out-of-pocket health expenditure, worsened, coupling higher taxes with increased health services devolution. The result of these developments would be a moribund tendency at both individual and communal levels, which motion both would likely resist, a resistance potentially expressed in electoral terms. Increasing devolution would also heighten latent tendencies toward adverse selection, a problem of which we currently only moderately have. These issues are not those we could sidestep. Indeed, the OECD, of which Canada is a member recently warned that health spending keeps rising in OECD countries and, if not curbed, governments will have to raise taxes, reduce spending in other areas or make people pay more out of their own pockets to sustain their current healthcare systems[7]. OECD Health Data 2006 revealed the faster growth in health spending than GDP in every OECD country other than Finland from 1990 to 2004, 7% of GDP on average across OECD countries in 1990, 8.8% and 8.9% in 2003 and 2004, respectively. Most of these countries financed healthcare via taxes, 73% on the average publicly funded in 2004. With medical technologies and population aging projected to put additional financial strain healthcare budgets in these countries down the road, one cannot overemphasize prudence in health spending rather than increasing devolution, to ensure sustainable health systems financing. In other words, we should aim to reduce both the public and private share of health spending by making the achievement of the dual healthcare delivery objectives (DHDO) our strategic intent. Public share of health spending keeps increasing in countries including Canada, but so is private payments for health, healthcare financed by private insurance, and directly out of the pocket, the latter a key source of financing in some OECD countries, particularly where private health insurance is low, 51% in Mexico in the 2004, the highest among OECD countries, for example. Private health insurance, money insurance firms pay out for health services, constitutes just about 6% of total health spending among OECD countries on the average, 10 to 15% of overall spending in Canada. With devolution would the roles private payments for health in Canada play increase, and would increase, out-of-pocket expenses were financing from private insurance to be low, due to adverse selection, for example, the combined effect of which would be to compromise the overall health Canadians, further worsening the 'wait lists' problem, as increased morbidity results in increased service utilization. These issues bring to the fore, the potential contributions to the prospects and challenges that the Canadian health system would confront of the changing dynamics of the public versus private financing of health in the country.

No doubt, this issue continues to feature prominently in the healthcare delivery landscape. With healthcare consumers likely, to choose insurance coverage based on anticipated need for the covered items, the likelier would persons want coverage for a particular item, and more of it too, having it, the higher the anticipated need for the item, than would someone who does not think he/she would need coverage for that item. This 'adverse selection,' could upset health risk pooling in the insurance arena, younger healthier individuals more inclined to purchase for example, high deductible plans, typically less generous than traditional, comprehensive plans, toward which latter persons likely to need coverage for long-term chronic diseases treatment, for example, with likelier less out-of-pocket spending saving on premiums buying high deductible plans, would gravitate. This explains why in general, high-deductible plans tend to be cheaper. However, with the potential for high deductible and customary, comprehensive plans ending up with skewed numbers of healthy and ill enrollees, respectively, the implications for high deductible plans versus other plans for claims costs and possibly premiums, with the latter not adjusted to show differences in enrollee risk between plans, could be dire. This is because the significant slanting of health spending, with a minute percentage responsible for a disproportionate share of spending in a given year, what might appear to be small differences in the numbers of 'high-cost' enrollees in a plan, high-deductible, customary, or other plans could significantly hike or decrease claims and plan costs due to 'adverse selection.' The more we devolve coverage in Canada therefore, the more Canadians would be liable to experience 'adverse selection,' making more comprehensive plans less generally affordable as persons anticipating the need for chronic long-term treatment, even if only a few, buy such policies, thereby hiking their costs, claims, hence premium, making them unaffordable to many who otherwise might also want it. These developments would eventually increase the numbers of the unhealthy, some of the illnesses and their complications covered by Medicare, swelling patronage at public health facilities, increasing 'wait times,' increasing healthcare costs, and spending. This scenario is even more likely to happen with the country's population aging, and the need for long-term management of chronic diseases likely to escalate, these developments potentially likely compounded by the fact that private funds seem to feature more prominently in purchasing medications, whose costs especially in treating chronic diseases could be quite high. This is more so, compared to, for funding hospital or ambulatory care, for example, as publicly financed insurance programs in general tend not to cover medications as robustly as do these other services, a situation which more devolution would further worsen. Among OECD countries for example, public coverage of spending on drugs was lowest in Mexico (12%), the United States (24%), Poland (37%) and Canada (38%) in 2004, compared to over two-thirds of medication expenditure publicly funded in countries such as Austria, France, Germany,

Spain and Sweden[7]. These issues simply mean that we should seek instead of tax hikes or increased devolution, for examples, other options in ensuring the provision of accessible and qualitative health services efficiently and cost-effectively, in effect pursuing the achievement of the dual healthcare delivery objectives (DHDO,) aggressively too. With adverse selection able to significantly influence claims cost and premiums, even with relatively minor changes in enrollment, as insurers predicate premiums on claims experience, or even on anticipated claims, Canada cannot afford the consequences of the disruption in access to care that would result with increasing provincial/territorial devolution of health services, including increased 'wait times.' The knock-on effects of these developments could be devastating not just for the country's health services, but also for its economy. The country would need to invest on research efforts to understand better the extent to which health jurisdictions could devolve services within the context of the Health Canada Act, and its guiding principles, to which all provinces and territories must legally subscribe, including researches on differences on health of the various health plans available in the private health sector. This is necessary considering the potential effects of these issues on the overall health of Canadians and the country's economy. Thus, as part of the country's efforts to ensure the accessibility to health services both within and outside Medicare, ensuring which is, as noted earlier, crucial to the health of the country in many respects and its sustenance, we should be interested in and be ready to collaborate with issues pertaining to health in all sectors of the country's economy. Thus, in addressing health issues, including the 'wait times' issue, we should appreciate the interconnectedness of these issues, health and non-health alike, and adopt equally multifaceted approaches to the solutions to these problems. Healthcare delivery is going to continue even more along the present multidimensional path in the years ahead, effective solutions to problems confronting it, inevitably going to demand a thorough understanding of these various issues. Taking cognizance of the importance of all Canadians being healthy is therefore, a cardinal underlying principle that must still guide us in the organization and delivery of health services, more so as its link with the economy, via happiness for example, is critical. The assumptions in the C18th Jeremy Bentham made in proposing that the object of public policy be the maximization of the sum of happiness in society that led economics to study utility or happiness, thought measurable and comparable, in detail, have generated much controversy over the years. Incidentally, the ideas of Bentham also led to the assumption that versus the rich, the marginal utility of income was more for the poor hence income needs redistribution except the efficiency cost in so doing was excessive, assumptions Lionel Robbins challenged in his book the 'Nature and Significance of Economic Science (1932.)' The positive economics that resulted from this challenge rooted in Robbins idea that predicting someone's behavior only requires assuming that the person has an unwavering set of preferences or ends, which how it arose is not the business of economics, and the measurability or comparability of the happiness level, unnecessary, has been just as contentious. However, and although Robbins did not advocate public policy analysis within a formal economic framework, his was the time the behaviorist paradigm held sway in the psychology and by induction, the economics zeitgeist. Not only is the defectiveness of formal measures such as the GDP as sole premises of public policy evident, for example in peoples' happiness levels not in consonance with increases over the years in many countries in their GDP, the significance of well-being as determinants of national wealth, hence premises for policy formulation is increasingly backed by research evidence. This has rekindled interests in the idea of maximizing the sum of human well-being, which as we discussed earlier, constitutes an important element of utilitarianism that requires approaching from novel perspectives rooted in the analyses of an amalgam of issues dictated by ongoing flux in knowledge and practice in multidisciplinary domains. It is in fact the case that we could gain insights with significant policy implications measuring happiness, and determining its causes and variables that affect it, versus those obtainable via the customary economics approach of inferring valuation from behavior through revealed preference, for example. Such measures for example would enable us appreciate the full impact of unemployment, as being far more than the loss of income for example, the dent in the psyche of feeling unwanted just as, if not more important, the potential of that for compromising physical in addition to mental health difficult to ignore. This is more so not just in relation to this situation worsening the problems our health system confronts, such as the 'wait times' issue, and soaring health spending, but also regarding more fundamental issues such as not meeting the rights of individuals to survive, albeit indirectly, and perhaps more directly, compromising the country's economy. Thus, that we need to ensure that unemployment levels are as low as possible becomes clear, in a more profound way than using standard economic variables to evaluate the problems consequent upon unemployment. In other words, it might be easier to assume that taking care of loss of income consequent upon loss of job via social assistance check, is all that we need to do for example, whereas measures of happiness would indicate otherwise. It would indicate for examples that in addition, we need to focus on reduce unemployment, getting people on social assistance back into the labor force as much as possible, and ensuring jobs are more secure for those employed, among others. This example underscores the multiplicity of factors that are crucial for us to explore, and the interplay between them, in any serious efforts to address problems with our health system, such as the 'wait times' and other healthcare accessibility issues. Many would contend that it is difficult to assure jobs availability much more security, but we might have to weigh our options critically considering the aforementioned, and assign the appropriate weight to variables, changes in which could result in more profound effects than others could. It is thus, important not just work being available, but that it does not psychologically distress workers, hence be counter-productive, as the example of interns' work hours mentioned earlier, with its potential to worsen the 'wait times' issue, compromise the quality of service delivery, jeopardize the lives of both patients and doctors, shows. Indeed, Canadian employers recently identified work-related stress as the biggest threat to their workers' well-being, with over 78% reporting it as their top 'health risk concern[8]'. What is more, another recent poll an AP-Ipsos survey conducted in November 2006 showed that three of four Canadians reported sometimes stressed, or frequently so, about the same levels, Americans reported, jobs and finances the most nerve-racking of parts their lives[9]. Time availability and utilization are among the other factors experts blame for these stress levels, for examples, traffic jams in urban areas, defective public transportation in suburban areas, increasing costs of living and mortgages in urban forcing individuals into the suburbs, resulting less time for sleep and families. Besides again pointing to the multidimensional nature of health issues and the need for inter-sectoral collaboration in solving them, we should focus in particular on mental health, as mental illnesses constitute some of the worst causes of unhappiness. Projections of health care spending in Canada indicate it would reach $148 billion in 2006, an increase of $8 billion over 2005, noted the annual report of the Canadian Institute for Health Information (CIHI)[9], *National Health Expenditure Trends, 1975– 2006*,health spending outpacing inflation and population growth for ten consecutive years, but do we spend enough on mental health? Should we not in fact be vigorously pursuing the achievement of the dual healthcare delivery objectives in mental health services provision as part of our overall efforts to achieve these goals? What roles could the implementation and utilization of healthcare information and communication technologies on a pervasive scale in the mental health services, play in the achievement of these objectives? Considering the major role life events play in the onset and perpetuation of unhappiness, for example, could these technologies not play key roles in acute and long-term stress management, for example in the provision of crisis intervention services, and ongoing tele-cognitive behavior therapy, which both could help facilitate access to care and reduce 'wait times'?

With regard onsite mental health services, patient turnover is much higher in psychiatric units of general hospitals, intake often via the ER, than in psychiatric hospitals whose patients often have more severe illnesses such as schizophrenia, the average hospitalizations stays in these two types of hospitals, 16.9 and 148.5 days respectively, versus 7.2 days for hospitalizations for non-psychiatric diagnoses. Also based on the CIHI report, mood disorders, namely depression and bipolar disorders, were the commonest psychiatric disorders, responsible for hospital separations, the level of use of hospital mental health services defined in terms of separations, regardless of age groups, provinces and territories, although schizophrenic and psychotic disorders were responsible for the highest percentage of hospitalization days. Also significantly, 1 in 5 separations for mental illness in 2003-2004 had a comorbid substance related disorder[10]. As benign as these figures might look, they have major significance for policy formulations. Versus psychiatric hospitals, the 'wait times' issue for example, is more problematic in general hospitals, where the need for beds are often more acute, considering not just the higher patient turnover, but also the role comorbid substance related disorders play in these admissions. The CIHI report mentioned earlier also noted that more than one in three patients (37%) discharged from a general hospital, diagnosed with mental illness were readmitted within a year, versus 27% of all other patients. Could we not therefore ease the pressure on beds in these hospitals preventing these disorders in the first place, instituting policies that would establish the appropriate programs to achieve this goal? Should we not be investing more resources in substance use disorders as a long-term strategy to reduce the prevalence (the incidence or rate, and duration) of these disorders? There are cell phones for example that could alert individuals to their blood alcohol levels, essentially warning them to stop drinking. Should we not promote the use of such technologies for instance, which could reduce the prevalence of these disorders? Could we not deploy healthcare information and communication technologies more in our efforts at primary, secondary, and tertiary disease prevention, the prevention of diseases in the first place, their prompt diagnosis and treatments, and the establishment of the appropriate treatment, including rehabilitation to prevent their sequelae, respectively? When George Still first discussed the disorder now termed ADHD in 1902 in *The Lancet*, [11] we did not know that ADHD was not just a hyperactive disorder of childhood, that it is a constellation of symptoms including inattention and compromised impulse control. Nor did we know that a proportion of childhood cases of ADHD persist into adulthood. Progress in the knowledge of ADHD and its treatment means we are now able to better help children and adults with this disorder, whose potential consequences for affected persons and their families could be devastating, not to mention the implications of these consequences cumulatively for the country. We could indeed, achieve the same positive results for other psychiatric disorders, the need for investment in research efforts on all aspects of which could yield substantial dividends in the years ahead, hardly contentious. This contrasts sharply with the legendary tendency in many countries to place less emphasis on mental health and psychiatric disorders. This contrast magnifies significantly in the context of the increasing knowledge of the role that happiness plays in our lives. This is even more so considering that it could, in our being able to evaluate social welfare more realistically and to improve which, it enables us develop, effective policies. It is also counter-intuitive even if real that we are not placing enough emphasis on mental health services, the readmission rates mentioned earlier, clearly indicative of flawed outpatient, follow-up, and rehabilitation services, and perhaps our failure to stabilize these patients' mental status effectively for a variety of other reasons, for example, using less effective, albeit cheaper, medications. The costs implications of repeated hospitalizations, relative to ambulatory or domiciliary treatment, are likely grim, and the need for appropriate policy formulations on these issues, whose knock-on effects would likely reduce scarce healthcare resources, which might worsen accessibility to health services, including increasing 'wait times,' in the health and even other service areas. That the risk of readmission to general hospital for persons with a primary diagnosis of mental illness is higher the older the persons is, 26.5 per 100 and 38.7 per 100 for persons 0 to 14 years, and 65 years and over, respectively, also has policy implications. This is so, considering the increasing longevity of Canadians, and the likelihood of comorbid physical illnesses, often chronic among older persons, both likely to increase treatment and hospitalization costs, hence health spending, hence the need for us to address these issues urgently, including the primary, secondary, and tertiary prevention of mental illnesses. The CIHI report indicated that the risk of readmission was higher for persons with a primary diagnosis of personality disorder (45%), schizophrenia (41%), next. It showed no gender differences, readmission rates for women and men, (38.3% and 35.5%, respectively, and showed that readmission rates in a year increased the longer the duration of the initial general hospital stay, all which again, indicate the important issues on which we should focus. As noted earlier, mood disorders are the commonest causes of psychiatric admission, hence also important areas to focus on, more in light of new research findings indicating the involvement of depression in changes in a part of the brain called the hippocampus, which is not only stress-sensitive, but also mediates learning and memory. It is even the more important that we focus on mood disorders considering the potential significance for management and policy formulation of the common co-occurrence with depression of a variety of medical conditions such as diabetes, heart diseases, and arthritis, and their equally common origin in stress-related metabolic disturbances. That these efforts could no doubt, help in more effective treatment of, and hence in improving the well-being of individuals that have these conditions, and in reducing associated healthcare costs, hence health spending, somewhere in the process, improving accessibility to health services, including reducing 'wait times.' It might appear circuitous some of the routes by which we have arrived at the conclusion of 'wait times' reduction. However, this is the very aim we have tried to achieve in this discussion of the subject, to stress a different perspective to approaching the 'wait times' issue, one eclectic at once cohesive, a global view that underscores the interrelatedness of health issues. There is no gainsaying the likely increasing importance of such approaches to addressing other health issues confronting Canada, and indeed other countries, in the emerging healthcare delivery playfield. Without such a comprehensive approach to tackling the country's healthcare issues, we would likely be wasting precious time and other resources pursuing policies that at best would be partial solutions to complex problems that we could otherwise solve more effectively, efficiently, and comprehensively. In a world in which not just the link between health and economic growth and development is increasingly recognized, but also where competition among nations and their elements in every economic sector is also ever more intense, Canada could hardly afford the luxury of such wastage. The time for us to act to stop it, is right now. The 'wait times' issue is essentially an accessibility issue, and lack of or delayed access to health services runs counter to some of our most cherished values, including assuring the right to life. Besides denying this right directly, it also does indirectly by compromising our ability to achieve the dual healthcare delivery objectives (DHDO), which by eventually resulting in increased morbidity and mortality, increases healthcare costs and health spending. The more of our resources we spend on health, the less we have to meet our other needs, and worse still, we would not necessarily improve the health of Canadians, if we did not change our approach to addressing health issues confronting the country. In other words, we would only be perpetuating the flaws that led to increased health spending in the first place, and spending even more on health and cascading down a moribund path. The temptation by provinces and territories to increase taxes or devolve services would increase, both of which could only worsen the economy and the health of our peoples. Even if our goal were to expand Medicare to more Canadians by rationing health services, the experience in the U.S., with the Oregon Health Plan (OHP) is instructive[12]. Enacted in 1989 with federal government approval as a Section 1115 Medicaid demonstration project in 1993, many hailed OHP as a foremost state policy innovation then. However, something appeared to have gone awry with the plan, which critics allege now covers fewer persons and services, and the picture in other states that have adopted the plan, even grimmer, the removal of entire benefit areas and reductions in recipients' numbers, seemingly capricious hacks, not the balanced and explicit prioritizing that was OHP's goal. In fact, Medicaid expenditure ballooned from about $750 million to $1.7 billion from the biennium prior to adopting and the first of OHP, enrollment by just a third[13]. The point here is that regardless how finite our health budget is, we need to be wary of the long-term health and economic benefits of such budgetary caps. There is no doubt about the need for us to control health spending, but should we not be so doing via curtailing healthcare costs reducing disease prevalence, as opposed to, for example, not making required upfront investments on healthcare information and communication technologies that could help us achieve the dual health delivery objectives (DHDO)? Even if a parallel private health system eventually emerges on a large scale in the country, these investments would have improved the public health system to compete effectively with the private health system, making concerns about the potential adverse consequences of the latter on the former essentially redundant. Furthermore, the moderation of costs that would eventually result from the intense competition among private healthcare providers with the emergence of a parallel private health system would improve accessibility to health services in both sectors, if the public health sector had invested in the technological power play that would characterize this competition. This would ensure not just the viability of the public health system, which would find it easier to devolve services, rationalizing and prioritizing, as this would not compromise access to care, and the overall health of Canadians, and the country's economy, in fact, would do the exact opposite more resources available for programs in other sectors of the economy. The dimensions of accessibility to care that we need to examine are indeed, legion. This though, should not deter us from so doing, as it would be antithetical to our overall interests not to do so. Canada's prospects, but also challenges regarding its health systems could affect other sectors of its economy profoundly. We must understand this important interplay of the country's economic sectors, as this, ultimately, is the key to our country's survival, and continued progress. Not just policy makers need to know about these important links, but also the public, because as the more, the public knows about them, the easier would it be for it to appreciate the important role of each individual Canadian in the country's continued existence, and prosperity. We need to inculcate in all Canadians, the vision of a new Canada in a new world and a new age, and their stake in it its realization. At the end of the day, all of us have to participate in solving problems such as the 'wait times' issue. From such simple measures as being committed to our scheduled doctor's appointment, or ensuring we cancelled it in time enough for it not to disrupt the activities of the doctor's practice, to being rational in our utilization of health services, and in our conduct of our daily living, regarding the latter, for example, cultivating healthy habits, every little helps, literally. We should also, and not just doctors and healthcare professionals alone, be prepared to embrace the widespread implementation and utilization of healthcare information and communication technologies, and other measures that could help us achieve the dual healthcare delivery objectives (DHDO). Part of appreciating our potential to contribute to our efforts to meet our rights, including in particular that to life is acknowledging the need for setting such goals, and the benefits derivable from such technologies, and indeed, other measures in achieving them, and of course our contributions to these benefits materializing. There is no doubt that we would accept the challenges that confront our health system, and overcome, and that great Canada would emerge even greater in the end.

References

1. To Err is Human: Building a Safer Health System, Linda T. Kohn, Janet M. Corrigan, and Molla S. Donaldson, Editors, Committee on Quality of Health Care in America Institute of Medicine, National Academy Press, Washington, D.C. 2000

2. Crossing the Quality Chasm: A new health System for the 21st century, Committee on Quality of Health Care in America Institute of Medicine, National Academy Press, Washington, D.C. March, 2001

3. Leape, Lucian; Lawthers, Ann G.; Brennan, Troyen A., et al. Pr e-venting Medical Injury. Qual Rev Bull. 19(5):144-149, 1993.

4. Gagnon, Louise. Medical error affects nearly 25% of Canadians, Canadian Medical Association, vol. 171 (2), 20 July 2004, p. 123

5. *Physicians' Extended Work Shifts Associated With Increased Risk of Medical Errors That Harm Patients*. Press Release, December 12, 2006. Agency for Healthcare Research and Quality, Rockville, MD. Available at: http://www.ahrq.gov/news/press/pr2006/extshiftpr.htm Accessed on December 24, 2006

6. Tanne, JH. United States limits resident physicians to 80-hour working week BMJ 2003; 326: 468b

7. Available at: http://www.oecd.org/document/37/0,2340,en_2649_37407_36986213_1_1_1_37407,00.html Accessed on December 25, 2006

8. Available at:
http://www.theglobeandmail.com/servlet/Page/document/v5/content/subscribe?user_URL=http://www.theglobeandmail.com%2Fservlet%2Fstory%2FLAC.20061027.CAWELL27%2FEmailTPStory%2F&ord=1167258501216&brand=theglobeandmail&force_login=true Accessed on December 27, 2006

9. http://secure.cihi.ca/cihiweb/dispPage.jsp?cw_page=AR_31_E&cw_topic=31 Accessed on December 27, 2006

10. Available at:
http://www.cihi.ca/cihiweb/dispPage.jsp?cw_page=AR364_2006sum_e Accessed on December 28, 2006

11. Still GF. Some abnormal psychical conditions in children: the Goulstonian lectures. Lancet. 1902; 1:1008-1012.

12. Oberlander. J., Health Reform Interrupted: The Unraveling Of The Oregon Health Plan *Health Affairs*, doi: 10.1377/hlthaff.26.1.w96 (Published online December 19, 2006) Available at:
http://content.healthaffairs.org/cgi/reprint/hlthaff.26.1.w96v1.pdf Accessed on December 30, 2006

13. Available at:
http://content.healthaffairs.org/cgi/eletters/hlthaff.26.1.w96v1#1347 Accessed on December 30, 2006

A Political Philosophy of Health

The decision by Canada's Supreme Court on June 09, 2005, to uphold the argument of Dr. Chaoulli and George Zeliotis, in their appeal against prior rulings by two lower courts that delay in accessing Medicare, and legislation limiting access to private health services in Quebec, violated section 7 of the Canadian Charter of Rights and Freedoms, was monumental. The implications for health policy of the issue of hospital-acquired, or nosocomial, Methicillin-Resistant Staphylococcus aureus (MRSA) infections, responsible for the deaths, according to 2005 estimates, of 3000 individuals per year in the country[1], was a main political issue in the 2005 UK general elections. In a 2000 article in The New England Journal of Medicine Dr. Paul Lichtenstein and his colleagues concluded that, 'inherited genetic factors make a minor contribution to susceptibility to most types of neoplasms. This finding indicates that the environment has the principal role in causing sporadic cancer[2],'as opposed to genes, a conclusion at which many other researchers have arrived[3, 4, 5], and which, with prostate cancer risk higher Asians when they immigrate to North America, implicates environment and lifestyle-related factors in causing prostate cancer in the U.S., for example. This is not to say that genes play no role in the causation of cancers, although teasing out the precise interactions between the environment and genes in this process has proven somewhat enigmatic[7, 8], which puts such major projects as the Human Genome Project and the resultant International HapMap Project in new perspectives, as it does principles underlying health policy. What these three seemingly disparate issues have in common is there interface with the philosophical underlay of contemporary healthcare delivery. With some Canadian provinces such as British Columbia, Alberta, Ontario explicit about their interests in private health systems, and Quebec, compelled by law to allow its residents to access even health services that Medicare covers, in the private, for-profit health sector, some are convinced that it is a matter of time before Canada has a full-blown, second-tier, for-profit health sector. This will no doubt include those with significant, perhaps even exclusive, foreign investments, in keeping with the country's regional and global trade accords, developments which some contemplate with intense foreboding for Canada's Medicare. Dutch researchers in 2005 found MRSA in three pig farmers/family members and their pigs, raising serious nosologic and policy issues[9], the outcome of which some farmers would await with trepidation and health authorities in their jurisdiction, equally apprehensively, considering the practical implications of these infections classified eventually as zoonoses, for example, on health services delivery, and indeed, animal husbandry. Furthermore, how would multimillion-dollar-genomic projects fare in a paradigmatic shift in the zeitgeist with focus on the milieu rather than the gene, exploring disease causation as evidence mounts for the former, with likewise fewer for the latter? What could this portend for the interplay of forces in the health, pharmaceutical, chemical, and other industries, and in government, whose outcome essentially makes health systems work? In other words, to what extent could health function, if at all, without these forces aligning and operating in tandem, and is healthcare delivery therefore, in ethereal suspense, the opus of a complex of industrial cacophony, government the conductor? The three issues mentioned above exemplify the profound nature of present-day healthcare delivery, the variables attendant to each, pervasive, crisscrossing the entire spectrum of social, political, and economic activities, and domains. Moreover, that these characteristically fluid activities/milieus crucially drive healthcare delivery, that is in turn, typically the progenitor of the elements of stability of both, is anything but trivial. It is apt therefore to ponder the roots of the justifiably termed frenetic pace of both elements of this healthcare delivery and activities/domains dyadic vis-à-vis the future of either, on the one hand, and those of the potential outcomes of the intimately intertwined symbiotic between them, on the other. Thus, we need to consider both the domestic and global elements of healthcare delivery as both determine the pace and outcomes of the elements of its complements mentioned above, alone and in concert that potentially strongly influence healthcare delivery. Our approach then needs to be pragmatic and at once philosophical, not least as the revival of normative political philosophy by John Rawls in his 1971 book, a Theory of Justice, continues to raise significant questions regarding important pragmatic perspectives. These include considerations regarding for examples the place of Benthamnism in contemporary political policy issues, including those pertaining to healthcare delivery, or the relevance of methodological individualism construed in behaviorists versus psychological terms. The increasing evidence of the inadequacy of formal economic variables such as the Gross National Product (GNP) and of less formal ones such as aggregating happiness for example as a social welfare functions, both reminiscent of attempts in works such as Herbert Simon's Models of My Life, to acknowledge the limits of human rationality, is instructive. It is also that such works thus also acknowledge those of rational choice theory, yet not totally jettison but transform the idea into for example that of 'bounded rationality.' This is more so considering the general tendency in healthcare to place the patient at the center of the healthcare delivery universe, literally, with concepts such as consumer-driven and patient-oriented healthcare, and similar terms, encapsulating the convergent key principle, and the problems of the validity of applicable policy orientation in different health jurisdictions it spawns, given the potential for fundamental conflicts locating underpinnings, philosophical or otherwise for this principle. It raises the issue for example of the truth or otherwise of the short-term as opposed to long-term utility, or survivability value of our actions, for most, including health policies, in Piercean terms, versus for example, as for William James and others, those actions that contribute most good to the individual, not the community. Thus, the very question of the dialectic between the individual and the community arises, in particular regarding the potential transition from the former to the latter and vice versa of the consequences of our actions, favorable or adverse. Where would this tension for example lead us in resolving the anti-selection issues some might contend the anti-smoking policy measures several health jurisdictions now take involve, including smoking ban in public places, and in restaurants, bars, and other locations.

Besides raising questions characteristic of those the critics of rational choice

theory ask, it also does so, those regarding the potential for information asymmetry changing the dialectic mentioned above, and as some would insist essentially skewing the basis of policy formulation in the Piercean direction. Howbeit, could the very fact that information asymmetry exists, be the reason policy formulation should not result in such skewing, but should in fact be predicated on the effective operations of individual/community dyadic? What are the implications of these issues for health services funding, for example, in particular, on the roles of public vis-à-vis private funding, the potential for both to coalesce or co-exist, as contemporary healthcare delivery evolves within the framework of equally emergent and fundamental changes in the global 'body politic.' Could we as some contend refocus health insurance for example, interest now on catastrophic, rather than universal coverage, or should we rectify information asymmetry, and attempt to turn its challenges into prospects, if possible? With regard the latter, would this eliminate the problems that moral hazard creates for our health systems, both privately and publicly funded, and accessibility to them, both of which could, by worsening the health of individuals, and by extension, overall health of the community, adversely affect a country's economy, creating a roller-coaster knock-on, with potentially devastating consequences for all? Thus, not fostering rational decision making, for example, by not creating the enabling environment for not just appropriate information necessary for such decision making not being exclusive, via say, the widespread implementation and utilization of healthcare information and communication technologies, with all parties in any transaction adequately served, could indeed, be double-edged. So could also even failing, to appreciate the need so to do. On the one hand, we would be perpetuating the very exclusivity of information that creates adverse selection, and not helping provide valuable, potentially life-changing information that could obviate moral hazard, hurting the health system, and perhaps, the overall economy. On the other, we would be compromising the accessibility of individuals to health services, as premiums become increasingly unaffordable, or the system economically no longer viable as health spending skyrockets. Additionally, we would be creating the grounds for the worsening of these potential developments with every day delay recognizing the crucial and ultimately inevitable necessity to appreciate the need for and act on fostering such rational decision making at individual, community, government, and state levels, and indeed, in the public and private domains of a country's economy. Even if information asymmetry could potentially be Piercean-friendly, that such predilection, if unchecked, could be tantamount to an infringement of the fundamental right to life of an individual is arguably real. In other words, could we not, by our inaction or otherwise, rectifying information asymmetry, hence providing the basis for rational choice be in fact compromising the very existence of these individuals. By extension, could we not, that of the community, which latter, some could construe to mean compromising the right to life of those individuals, for example that do not engage in risky lifestyles, for who nonetheless, adverse selection, for example, has made access to health services impossible? Assuming that those individuals that engage in unhealthy lifestyles are in fact doing so as some means to installmental suicide, which itself is arguable, considering the tendency for motion, individual and collective, in the same direction, in the main of life, as opposed to death, the question whether we should let them do so is also arguable. This is not to mention that which the community, moribund taking these persons along implies, such as, essentially denying them the right to life.

These issues are clearly germane to the validity of the fabric of our healthcare policies. In the true pragmatist tradition, we could argue that what is true must contribute the most good for the longest term, albeit not necessarily that whatever works is only what is true. In particular, some would contend that political expediency requires pragmatic agility. Thus, that it would be politically naïve to ignore the practical consequences of the collective perspective, and indeed, action. The point however, is that such action has its roots in those of individuals, as noted above. This emphasizes the somewhat obscure aspects of the individual/community dyadic mentioned earlier, whose propensity to shake some of our most cherished values to their cores is humbling. An example of this is the inevitable need of the individual to seek the right to life, and the corresponding need of the community for the individual to seek that of the community to life, which the community in the main seeks, is hardly contestable.

This dynamics is most evident in the operations of a democracy, which indeed, most expediently motorizes an inevitable interplay inherent in which is the tendency of most persons to seek to live rather than to die. The pace of the achievement of this tendency is a function of the effectiveness and efficiency of the political economy, including that of a country's health system, itself the benchmark for the prospects of 'true' progress. The distinction between this type of progress and the 'spurious' could not be more evident in the sustainability of the progress of states in recent history, and would be even more so in that of the emerging picture of world economies over time. Thus, until human beings cede the running of the affairs of states to humanoids, or even straight-through mechanical devices perhaps called a different name than robots, when even arguments regarding the importance or otherwise of 'humanoid or robot capital' would likely emerge, the pivotal role of human capital remains unquestionable. This is so despite that some would argue that countries such as Botswana, have wangled their way to prosperity with relatively limited human capital. However, such examples do not nullify the fact that consideration of human capital is crucial in any equation on the prosperity of nations. In fact, they exemplify the stepwise evolution of sustainable development, and the need for such countries to fast track that of the development of their human capital, which they would need to sustain and perhaps improve their current levels of prosperity, and in the very extreme, and in the long term, their very survival in an increasingly hyper-competitive world. In other words, every country needs some measure of ongoing economic activities within their borders, and between them and other countries, human capital a critical aspect of these activities, and their long term continuity, the effective and efficient operations of these internal and external market and economic operations, and their sustainability, the hallmarks of 'true' prosperity. This highlights the importance of the institutions within these states, of which government and its various elements are important constituents, and of those that states have agreed upon to form that guide the conduct of international commerce. The importance of these institutions rests more though, in their roles in fostering or motorizing, even accelerating, the mechanisms, necessary for the realization of the objectives of the states in which they are to prosper, or put differently, to survive, and prosper. The corollary is thus true, that the lack of these institutions, or if present, their redundancy, or inadequacies in meeting the demands of the static and dynamic factors constantly impinging on them, could decelerate, even hinder, progress toward achieving these objectives, and could potentially lay bare the elements of spurious prosperity. It is therefore important for us to appreciate the requirements for not just progress, but of genuine, sustainable progress, a matter for ongoing across-board focus in countries determined to achieve these objectives, which in fact, all countries do, as it is inevitable not do otherwise. The question then is whether a country shifts gear, and does otherwise, which is possible, giving certain catastrophic circumstances, natural, and manmade, but whose probabilities, except of course in the former case could be increasingly dim in contemporary times. This is more likely so if we indeed, appreciated the various dimensions of health such as we have discussed thus, hence to for example, not continue to pollute our environment, considering as noted earlier, the significant role the environment plays in the causation of cancers.

There is no doubt about some individuals, groups of individuals, or even persons on state orders deliberately exercising the right to die, but this right or tendency toward death is mostly dormant in most persons, hence communities, until in persons, expressed in death due to old age or to disease. On the whole therefore, every country would inevitable have to create the enabling environment for the necessary institutions to thrive that would facilitate the efficient and effective functioning of the mechanisms crucial for economic growth and sustainable development, were its progress to be genuine and long-lasting. This implies that only countries that do so would have such enduring progress, those that do not, simply prolonging the unfolding saga of the interplay of the various elements that propel their human capital into an effective and efficient agent of progress. Grinding poverty, pervasive disease, compromised productivity, misery, and frustration, are all variables in such countries that would work their way, no matter how slowly into an implosion. This implosion would evolve ultimately in the direction of life, the more intense the hindrance, for example, occasioned by flawed government regardless of type, which itself implies absent or equally flawed institutions, the longer the delay, and more dramatic the implosion, which would, again, in the main be devoid of nosologic encumbrances. Contrariwise, the shorter the delay, the less dramatic the implosion, which would occur in any case in any society wherein the tendency toward life seems compromised, even if not as severely as perceived. This last statement is important with particular reference to developed countries, where some of these institutions need revamping in keeping with current requirements, an example, of such institutions being those pertaining to health and healthcare delivery. It also underscores the significance and indeed, applicability to all countries of the two most fundamental economic principles, namely that there will always be scarcity, so long as we are unable to meet all the needs of everyone, all the time, hence we would need to develop the means to allocate and use our scarce resources optimally. Thus, the perception of the efficient operations of the health systems in these countries is as important as the health systems in fact being so. This is more so considering the profound effects even minor hiccups in their operations could have on those of highly developed markets, the potential for capital flight, operational in seconds, with devastating consequences for the competitiveness of countries relative to competition. The prevention of such situations clearly require close attention to the health system, in the first place acknowledging that it is not perfect, and could never be, partly due to factors inherent in the system, such as the ever-changing knowledge base of medical practice, and indeed, of the healthcare information and communication technologies (ICT) and other technologies that power it. This is not to mention changes in other aspects of the transactions resulting in health care delivery, for examples, in management and accounting practices, and regarding accountability, and operational transparency. It is also partly due to the equally dynamic external milieu of healthcare delivery, including in the socio-political, economic, and ethico-moral domains within, and indeed, outside the country. Considering that no health system could ever be perfect, which corresponds with the economic principles mentioned earlier, we then need to find ways to make your health system as close to perfection as possible at any given time. This implies that we need to make it as efficient and as effective as possible, in effect to strive to achieve the dual healthcare delivery objectives (DHDO). This means that we aim for a health system that delivers qualitative health services, and simultaneously to reduce health spending, which are the hallmarks of effectiveness and efficiency. Furthermore, this means that we would have to subject all the elements of the operations of our health system to scrutiny, perpetually, to determine its 'weak' points and 'missing links' and the appropriate ways by which to rectify the problems. For this to happen, every health system has to conduct ongoing process cycle analyses on identified issues and problems, and on existing processes, problematic or not, in the form of periodic audits, and quality evaluation exercises. These analyses and exercises would reveal aspects of the health system that need improving, even expunging, for the entire system to work better, and for us to be able to achieve these dual goals. Implicit in these exercises is the underlying role of policy, the development, and implementation of which are essential for us also to pay attention.

Also assumed is that the role of government, the essential organ of state, which in democracies, represents the will of the majority, hence the tendency mentioned earlier of which to seek life rather than death, and which in other governmental arrangements in time it also would, increases the stakes regarding formulating and implementing the appropriate health and related policies. This places many governments in democracies in particular in a quagmire regarding the role, nature, and extent of the political philosophy and economic paradigms to underpin such policies, a potentially explosive situation as health jurisdictions drift amid incoherent policies, with costs implications. The example of certain stupendous debts that states and local governments in the U.S., have piled up, illustrate this point. About US$1.9 trillion in bonds debts, under-funding of pension plans up to US$700 billion, government employees' retiree health plans are also grossly under-funded, according to some estimates for twenty-seven jurisdictions, by $1.4 trillion countrywide[10]. The implications of this state of affairs for taxpayers is dire, the need for key policy reorientation in benefit plans and other government spending no doubt urgent. This is more so considering the projected increase in what these benefits would cost as large numbers of baby-boomers retire, and the population ages, a scenario that applies to other developed countries, for examples Canada, and the U.K. It would be reasonable to expect living standards of retirees to fall and their health to depreciate in these countries, were these debts to continue to rise, considering the limits to which tax increases could go without backfiring on the economy plunging it into a potentially vicious cycle of decadence. Indeed, the effects of not addressing this issue on living standards would be more pervasive, also more dramatic for other vulnerable members of society, widening the inequality gap that currently exists, which many governments struggle to close, testing our commitment to, perhaps even our appreciation of the roots of the need to close this gap, and not widen it.

The additional problems of implementation costs of policies that emerge even appreciating these roots further highlight the significance of the roots, and the need to upgrade them to meet contemporary challenges. This perhaps is an important reason for the wide acclaim in the philosophical zeitgeist of the efforts of such thinkers as John Rawls mentioned earlier that keep even seemingly forgotten ideas in perspective given new realities in which contextually and in association with other ideas, they might reveal hitherto cryptic yet profound insights into addressing current problems. Thus, many policy recommendations go unimplemented for costs reasons, which itself underscores the points made earlier about the scarcity of resources and the need for their rational allocation and utilization, the preference of governments for implementation then, often predicated on precedents and are characteristically incremental. This brings to the fore in our efforts to ensure the chances of evidence-based policy advice transitioning to implementation, including the probability of establishing new institutions, and strengthen current ones, the need to appreciate the importance of presentation, which in feasible, controllable, and attractive manner, given the prevailing economic, socio-political, and organizational milieus, likelier achieves this goal. This, itself highlights the relevance of focus on the technical underpinnings of the eclectic philosophical roots for examples, pragmatism within a utilitarian umbrella, of contemporary healthcare delivery, in the conduct of the latter. This is more so as is the case with the 1988, Sir Donald Acheson-led, independent inquiry into inequalities in health in the UK, which government explicitly asked to keep 'within the broad framework of the government's overall financial strategy,' a reflection of tight budgetary inclinations that effectively compromised the specification/costing, let alone implementation of aspects of the suggested policies. Incidentally, the third recommendation in the Acheson report specified the need for policies to 'reduce income inequalities and improve the living standards of households in receipt of social security benefits, ' and to increase benefits in cash or in kind to reduce 'poverty in women of childbearing age, expectant mothers, young children and older people[11]'. Considering that an earlier inquiry[12], led by Douglas Black, made similar recommendations, and had also confronted costs challenges, the difficulties estimating the influence of key drivers in specific policies on structural trends in living standards inequalities, as we should, is not far to seek. Yet, that we need to address issues such as child benefits, and single parent stipends, in Canada, for example, in keeping with the core values of its peoples, is doubtless, and suggests the need to weigh the benefits versus costs of not doing so. This is important were we to close the inequality gap, including in healthcare delivery, in the country. Indeed, if we did not do so, we could be at risk of significant potential adverse consequences for healthcare delivery, and indeed, by compromising access to health and to education for affected children for example, significantly deplete the stock of the country's expertise pool, which would also negatively affect its economy. The potential long-term consequences of failures in this regard for the country's economic development are obvious, as indeed, should be those of failures in formulating and implementing policies that could improve health in general, and if not, research evidence backs it up, even in developed countries[13, 14, 15]. In 2001, the Commission on Macroeconomics and Health noted the negative effect of ill health on economic growth levels in underprivileged countries[13], and that investment in a number of essential healthcare initiatives would result in significant economic growth. Studies have shown similar findings for rich countries[14] in whose current economic wealth the accrued benefits of preceding health status play a key role, about 30% of UK's economic growth from 1790 to 1980 due to improved health and dietary intake[14], for example. Indeed, a study in ten industrialized nations up to the mid-1990s showed improved health increased economic growth rate by roughly 30%[15]. More recent studies not using life expectancy, an excellent predictor even superior to education, of economic growth in developing countries[16], but which varies little among developed countries, but such measures as decrease in cardiovascular mortality, which varies significantly among industrialized countries, as a veritable predictor of ensuing economic growth, have arrived at similar conclusions[17]. There is no doubt that more of such studies would not only facilitate policy formulation, but also government's obligation to their implementation, or would they? The controversy over the validity of the concept of social welfare maximization, a carryover of utilitarianism into mainstream modern economics by Theil[18], and Tinbergen [19], which classical welfare economics rejects, despite enabling the derivation of optimal policies numerically, and offering an overall as opposed to several outcome measures in the use of life satisfaction or happiness, for example, is telling. Yet, we could hardly dismiss off-hand these objections, for examples on grounds such as difficulty of the measures being cardinal, and individual judgment being comparable, among others.

Even more subtle and perhaps more crucial with regard this same measure for example are the issues of hedonic adaptation and aspiration treadmill, the short-lived experiences of happiness reported due to adaptation of many to live events changes, and the modification in aspirations that these live events occasion, respectively. These phenomena raise, crucial policy issues in for examples how we recompense different individuals with different adaptive capacities that have experienced similar life events and effects, or should an individual be able to access whatever standard of public health services they could organize with how much funds they could spare, including for example, being able to circumvent hospital 'wait lists'? Then there is the 'benevolent dictator' concept that discards social welfare maximization on grounds of its ignoring or replacing existing political institutions and processes, hence government, keener on voter preferences revealed in polls and elections, either discountenances it or lacks the motivation to implement it. Whereas, that even dictators must consider the popular will to perpetuate their hegemony attests to the power of the people, not to mention the potential for politicians and interests groups to pander, with what, even social welfare maximization, has electoral leverage, is also instructive. Although, this is an aspect of the criticisms of the use of customary economic indicators such as the GNP, and unemployment for examples, at the very least, it suggests a certain inclination toward an inevitable motion in the direction of the collective right to life mentioned earlier, which not even agenda-driven, interest-group laden, democratic political processes can ignore. Thus, we all cannot ignore the need for qualitative healthcare delivery for all, and indeed, and cannot afford to fail to act on important determinants of health such as tackling poverty and closing the inequality gap. Efforts are ongoing in Canada to reduce the inequality gap in access to health for example via the activities of Canada Health Infoway Inc., which along with its partners are currently managing more than 150 projects, aimed at delivering electronic health record (EHR) solutions for Canadians[20]. Since the First Ministers of Canada's federal, provincial and territorial governments agreed in 2001 to utilize the country's technological capacity to improve healthcare in Canada via a Canada-wide health infostructure based on a universal framework that would support health providers, managers, and patients in effective decision making on healthcare, Canada Health Infoway has been active nationwide. With $1.2 billion in investment capital in hand, Infoway has approved over $700 million in electronic health record projects in all jurisdictions across the country, over the next year planning to approve another $335 million in new project investments, and by March 31, 2007 would have approved for specific projects about $1 billion (85%) of the investment capital[20]. With clinics, hospitals, pharmacies, community health centers, and other health portals connected access to health services would improve, even in currently underserved areas, and the quality of care delivered would improve, as would the burden of diseases lessen, and would the country become more economically vibrant, or would it? The need for this question arises for various reasons, not least the nature, and type of intervention and by which level of government in the implementation and use of healthcare ICT, including its pervasiveness. This latter highlights another reason for the question, that of the incompleteness of the connectivity link with the patients, and other healthcare stakeholders, for example, insurance firms, not included. Let us quickly illustrate this with say a national recall of a particular medication, the EHR we have implemented enabling the physician to access the full medication profile of affected patients, and contact them promptly to terminate use of the drug. Would that contact not be speedier the EHR detecting this recall, identifying the affected patients, and alerting them, and their physicians, all electronically, and could this not potentially save more lives, and money than carried out non-electronically, for example via snail mail? Thus, we still have work to do regarding our efforts to utilize EHR in healthcare delivery, not just in promoting the adoption of these technologies also by healthcare consumers. Indeed, we also need to promote the adoption and use of these technologies by our doctors and other healthcare professionals, who even recent studies comparing the use of these technologies in some developed countries by doctors, showed are way behind in so doing[21].

An international survey, for example that revealed conspicuous differences in primary care practice among developed countries, highlight the importance of having national policies in support of primary care, although in fact, we should have such policies to support healthcare delivery in general[21]. This survey showed that U.S. primary care physicians (PCP) are some of the unlikeliest to have extensive healthcare ICT or quality-based payment incentives; to provide access to after-hours care; and the likeliest to note problems that their patients have problems paying for care[21]. Also according to this survey, just 28% and 23% of U.S and Canadian doctors, respectively, reported using electronic medical records (EMRs), versus their use by most doctors in the Netherlands (98%), New Zealand (92%), the U.K. (89%), and Australia (79%). The survey also showed that Canadian and U.S. doctors are also unlikeliest to have decision support systems (DSS), such as the computerized alerts about potentially harmful drug doses or interactions, mentioned above, with just 10% and 23% of Canadian and U.S doctors receiving such alerts. In Netherlands, for example, 93% of doctors do, and 40% in Germany, do. Additionally, two of five Canadian and U.S. doctors reported finding it 'very difficult' or 'impossible' to know patients past due for testing or preventive care, whereas one of five or fewer do in the other countries. These figures no doubt underscore the need for more efforts in promoting the use of healthcare ICT, which could, as noted earlier facilitate the achievement of the dual healthcare delivery objectives (DHDO), among not just primary care doctors, but all doctors, in general, not to mention among patients too. There is no doubt that costs are important obstacles to implementing these technologies, but with, among others, the recent announcement by a Cambridge-based, UK firm Plastic Logic that it will build the world's first factory to produce plastic electronic devices, including plastic chips, we might be about to witness a new era in the computer chip industry[22]. Indeed, this might be so in the rest of the computer industry with the evolution of novel technologies such as electronic paper, as unlike silicon, the manufacture of plastic circuits requires the use of simple printing techniques. Perhaps even more importantly, besides widening the scope of the use of computers and related technologies in healthcare delivery, plastic circuits would significantly reduce the price of chips by as much as 90% and of healthcare ICT and consumer electronic goods, facilitating their widespread diffusion in the health sector among various stakeholders, including doctors and patients. Plastic Logic, a Cambridge University spin-off, which has been making plastic electronic devices since 2000, intends to build its factory in Dresden, Germany, for which it has secured $100m (£50.6m) venture capital funding, and is developing 'control circuits' that would be behind screens on electronic displays. Its electronic circuitry for 'electronic paper' displays would be able to store texts for several books for example, the potential to be more commonly used that paper in future, real, projected market worth for plastic electronics, US$30billion by 2015[22]. With the factory expected built in 2008, and billed to be able to manufacture one million control circuits, and the market expected to balloon to 41.6 million units in 2010, plastic chips and electronic paper are likely going to have profound effects on healthcare delivery also here in Canada. It would in fact also be the case, in other sectors of the country's economy. Progress in healthcare ICT would doubtless be a driving force in healthcare delivery in Canada, and we should exploit the opportunities that these technologies offer. Nonetheless, we could not claim to be so doing most of our doctors and other healthcare providers, and healthcare consumers not in the nationwide EHR 'loop' so to say. In fact, we risk our efforts in implementing these nationwide electronic health networks not achieving the desired objective, at least not in full, not involving as a matter of policy, all healthcare stakeholders in their evolution. As we queried earlier though, this brings to the fore issues regarding government interventions, why, their nature, extent, and at what levels. Should governments in Canada, and which, federal, or provincial and territorial, for examples, offer payments or other incentives to doctors for managing chronic disease, or meeting clinical targets, or should they not? Should doctors receive incentives for fostering preventive care, or engaging in other quality improvement activities, utilizing healthcare ICT for example? In the U.K for example, 95% of doctors receive, or could receive, financial incentives for improved performance[21]. Which governmental level should be actively involved in and to what extent, promoting the adoption of healthcare ICT among doctors and other healthcare professionals? Considering the importance of chronic disease management in particular with the likely increase in the prevalence of these conditions with the country's population aging, that a high percentage of doctors in all countries, 25% to 30% or over, in the survey mentioned above,

Germany, 7%, excepted, indicated their ill-preparedness to manage patients with multiple chronic diseases, is telling. Should the federal government actively participate in policy formulation and implementation to promote the use of healthcare ICT for example, and other measures proven to improve the prognosis of these disorders, in their management? In what issues and to what extent should Ottawa participate regarding policy?

Recently, the French government announced plans to make housing a legally enforceable right, via its Prime Minister, Dominique de Villepin, who indicated the imminent presentation of a housing bill to the cabinet on January 17, 2007, apparently in response to increased pressure to assist the homeless[23]. The government plan, commencing late 2008, would make the right to housing applicable to homeless people, impoverished workers and single mothers, all persons living in slums to benefit from the same right with effect from 2012, the plan requiring the construction of 120,000 new homes every year up to 2012. This new law would place housing in the same legal category as education and health in French legislation, the issue a key election issue in the country's forthcoming Presidential election in April 2007. It not only highlights the important connection between the right to life, and the rights that follow from it, or some would argue how to view interests posing as rights, or that could have the status of considering the exigencies of the times. The point in fact is that of the potential for being homeless to compromise the right to life, or put differently, the right to having a home being sine qua non to the right to life. It is not only counterintuitive to reject these notions, but that becomes even more evident considering the transition, or motion of rights from the individual to the collective or community levels and vice versa. Would some people being homeless or denied the opportunity of having a home serve the best interests of the right to life of the community? These questions, which we could extend to the potential of compromising the right to life of the community, resulting in compromising the economy, and further making it even harder for the homeless to survive, and indeed, for the community too, also raise another key issue, that of redistribution, which governmental level handles it, and why. Some would contend for example, as the case in France mentioned above shows that the federal government must handle such policies as welfare, as provinces would steer clear wary of becoming trapped in a welfare vicious cycle. This is so with redistribution to the homeless and poor soars demand for it from different categories of the poor, for example, from the almost deprived or poor, then from those somewhat deprived, next from the working deprived, et cetera, the enormous and excess intra-middle-class redistribution that follows, veritable economic warp drivers. Many experts believe the provinces would fare better, unlikely to be able to stomach excess redistribution, not least because of the financial burden of responsibilities for unemployment benefits, minimum wages, and other welfare programs, they already bear, not to mention for health services provision. The question remains though if provinces and territories should handle all the policies necessary to ensure that all the initiatives necessary to foster the achievement of the dual healthcare delivery objectives (DHDO), which essentially leads to the achievement of the right to life at both individual and community levels. If they should not, in which ones should the federal government be an active participant? For example, should it be in setting minimum technical standards for the nationwide implementation of healthcare information and communication technologies, to facilitate interoperability of legacy or current systems? Should it be fostering the pervasiveness of these technologies in a variety of other ways, setting other standards, for example, privacy standards, or those regarding minimum acceptable 'wait times' limits? The provinces and territories are essentially in charge of healthcare delivery in their jurisdictions. Yet, some of the goals of healthcare delivery are not limited to jurisdictions, but concern the entire country, its overall health, economic productivity, even survival. It is therefore reasonable to suggest that the federal government be actively involved in matters of health, and indeed, is, for example, via Canada Health Infoway mentioned earlier, and its various other initiatives, and via the activities of a variety of other agencies, even if indirectly. Some would say for example that the federal government essentially disapproving of Alberta's proposed 'Third Way,' Health plan, which would accommodate coexisting private healthcare delivery in the province, eventually led to its demise, which some would consider, 'over-involvement' in matters under provincial jurisdiction. These issues make constructing limits of federal involvement in a variety of health and welfare-related matters among others, contentious, some even considering the debate redundant pitched firmly in the opposing camps.

It is possible to see why the federal government should want to establish minimum standards for 'wait times.' Across the country, for example, considering that every Canadian should in accordance with the preservation of the right to life, have access to identical levels of qualitative health services is clear. However, it is also easy to see why stipulating these levels with any measure of precision would be futile, considering not just the variations in the availability of professionals for a particular specialty for example, the distribution of these professionals, and the accessibility to services otherwise. This is not mentioning the availability, and sophistication of healthcare ICT that could facilitate access to professional care, and improve its quality. Would it therefore not be more realistic for the population a health jurisdiction serves to be an active participant in the processes involved in defining the various dimensions of the health jurisdiction's 'wait times' issue and devising the best solution to them, based on the realities of that health jurisdiction? Could this not be within the context of the guiding principles of the Canada Health Act, for example? This issue brings to the fore the important role of information in the entire process of not just improving our health services, but also every aspect of our lives, of the Canadian economy, and of the country's prosperity, and indeed, of its survival. In other words, both provincial and territorial governments in Canada, and indeed, the federal government should consider the need for the populace to have information, crucial. A thorough appreciation by the Canadian public of the important role of healthcare ICT for example in improving our health system would facilitate the widespread diffusion of these technologies, which is critical to completing the connectivity link mentioned earlier that would make our substantial investments in EHR technologies via Canada Health Infoway mentioned above, achieve its intended goal. Thus, we need to promote education at all levels, which embraces information acquisition and that of a variety of the skills and 'attitudes' that would ultimately work for the betterment of each person, and the community at large. Now, perhaps we should emphasize this point with the results of recent researches that indicate that the single social factor consistently linked to longevity in every country where examined is education[24], more significant than race, income, even health insurance, and indeed, than many of the factors popularly deemed critical to living long. It is common knowledge that the distribution of longevity is not even in every society, certain groups with a tendency to live longer than others do. The pivotal role that education plays in longevity compared to for example, giving people more Social Security income, or in fact people having less of it, suggests that while it might be okay to give Canadians more of such money for other reasons, health is certainly not a major reason to do so. This calls for policy reorientation in Canada regarding the issue of education in relation to health and longevity, and as we have noted, what role each governmental level would play in this regard, considering the importance of the matter. These studies also call for a new approach to policy formulation on ensuring that our youths attend and remain in school, as studies show a significant link between a few additional years in school and not just more years of life, but also significant improvement in health later in life as the individual ages. Thus, by focusing policy on education, we would not just be improving the literacy levels of society, which has implications for economic productivity, but also helping to improve health, and in fact, preserve the right of individual Canadians to life. This issue underlines the complexity of the issues that we need to address, both in the health and non-health domains, in seeking to improve health services provision, the overall health of Canadians, and that of the country's economy. It is clear that we could improve health by focusing on education policy, including adult education and the provision of knowledge and skills required in the efficient conduct of everyday life. Thus, this would help us redress the information asymmetry problem pervasive in the health sector, making the healthcare consumer better able to take discerning measures regarding health. An example would be as simple a situation as appreciating the potential costs implications in, and the disruption of services that could hinder the access of someone else to crucial and urgent medical attention, frivolously skipping doctors' appointments. Another would be to reject smoking, which significantly reduces one's life span based not just base on the knowledge that it does, but also on a deeper understanding of the link between that person's life, and that of the community, which organic link now transcends that person's life.

The recognition at deeper cognitive and emotional levels that it includes those

of his or her parents, siblings, cousins, uncles and aunts, and indeed, that of everyone else, would be likelier with higher education and more information raising the insight level of the person. This would likely be more so considering also the link between having family and social networks and health and longevity. This link between education and health/longevity raises some key questions about the future direction of government policies in Canada on education and health, vis-à-vis children, single parents, parents in general, our concept of education in general, for example the emphasis on brick-and-mortar as opposed to distance/online education for example, and continuing adult education, among others. While the relationship between education and health might not be a direct causal one, at least not all the time, it remains solid, nonetheless. This is also not a matter of investing in one more than do in the other, as both constitute a symbiotic dyadic. We need policy changes that would essentially result in children going to school and remaining there for as long as possible. Here again, the issue of what role government has to play in this regard becomes crucial, as does what governmental level should play any role. Could we for example achieve our goal making schooling compulsory to higher than age 16 years, as currently is the case, harmonizing high school grades, generally 9-12 currently, but 8-12 in Vancouver, and 7-11 in Quebec, and should we use other measures to ensure the achievement of this goal? What role should french education play in the rest of Canada, and English in Quebec, in relation to the bilingual official status of the country, and indeed, should we group schools based on religion as used to be the case, run by school boards, or by some other agencies, and should there be federal government involvement of some sorts? Should we establish other policies in place of making schooling compulsory that have the potential to promote school attendance more effectively, and on the free will of young persons, considering that many young persons still do not attend school or drop out of school even with our current compulsory school policies? These questions are in keeping with the need to tease out the philosophical roots of our policies in different domains of economic and social activities mentioned earlier in our discussion. In other words, should our approach to policy not predicate on the role an appreciation of the interplay of individual/community dyadic by all would play in this regard? Should this be so even if several research studies looking at the effects of education showed that attending school for longer periods resulted in better health and longer lives[24,25,26]? The issue then from a pragmatic viewpoint is whether there is need for compulsion, or not, to achieve the desired objective of overall health improvement at the individual and community levels, and whether we should look at systemic changes that would promote a life-long interest in the knowledge acquisition among Canadians, and not just education up to high school. There is no doubt about the benefits of decreasing mortality in many countries for improved health for those alive, with individuals not just living longer, but also better and healthier[27]. Research also showed that and with income fixed, longevity still increased, life expectancy in China in 2000, 72 years, that in the U.S in 1970, despite having equivalent income levels to that of the latter in the 1880s, buttressing the fact that income alone does not increase longevity. Other studies measured the value of fall in mortality, including that of improved health for those alive, one showing that the yearly value of increased longevity was about 50% of national income measured via customary variables between 1970 and 2000[28]. These studies underline the complexity of the association between health and social status, although it is evident from research that the much of the causative direction of the link between health and income is that of the former causing the latter rather than the other way round. Experts have noted that the direct advantageous effect that education has on health is most likely responsible for this causative direction, even if the precise nature of the mechanisms involved remains obscure, and the subject of ongoing research[24]. These issues highlight the need for us to continue in our quest to make our health services best able to provide qualitative healthcare to Canadians, efficiently and cost-effectively. The researchers mentioned above point to the importance of the health and income dyadic that we have talked so much about in this discussion, and that of education in its operations, in particular in how improved overall health could improve the country's economy. The relationship is evidently symbiotic although the direction is more toward health improving the economy, than the reverse, which does not mean that income does not improve health as some studies of 'health inequalities' or gradient, showed that individuals with low-income live shorter lives than those with high-income[29]. According to the U.K's Office of National Statistics, 2005, unskilled male manual workers in England and Wales in 1997-2001, would likely live 8.4 years less from birth than do professionals do for example[30]. This, again points to the importance of education to income, and in being important to health, which effect does not fade, its significance as the link between both. It also therefore, emphasizes the importance of rectifying information asymmetry in the health sector, part of what an overall educational policy would achieve, which also underscores the need for us to focus on promoting the widespread adoption, implementation, and utilization of healthcare information and communication technologies, which incidentally should feature prominently in our general educational polices, by all healthcare stakeholders. These technologies would facilitate the acquisition of both the knowledge and skills necessary to take appropriate decisions, for example, recognizing danger, planning, and delaying gratification, not being able to do so, limited education no doubt fosters, considering that inadequately educated people are more likely to smoke[31]. With more financially challenged individuals likelier to lack health insurance, in the U.S., for example, and likely here in Canada, private health insurance, they would likelier be unable to receive necessary health services, which might compromise their ability to work and earn income, plunging them into a vicious cycle of worsening health. If we considered the effect of this situation on the aggregate of health, how our economy could progressively worsen is not far to seek. This issue points to the need for Canadians to have access to qualitative health services, and for its health jurisdictions to work toward achieving the dual healthcare delivery objectives

(DHDO), hence contribute not just to improving the health of Canadians, but also assuring their right to life, and the survival and progress of Canada.

References

1. Johnson AP, Pearson A, Duckworth G (2005). 'Surveillance and epidemiology of MRSA bacteraemia in the UK'. J Antimicrob Chemother 56 (3): 455-62.

2. Lichtenstein, P., Holm, N.V., Verkasalo, P.K., Iliadou, A., Kaprio, J., Koskenvuo, M., Pukkala, E., Skytthe, A. and Hemminki, K. (2000) Environmental and heritable factors in the causation of cancer — analyses of cohorts of twins from Sweden, Denmark, and Finland. N. Engl. J. Med., 343, 78–85.

3. Whittemore AS, Kolonel LN, Wu AH, et al. Prostate cancer in relation to diet, physical activity, and body size in blacks, whites, and Asians in the United States and Canada. J Natl Cancer Inst 1995; 87:652-661.

4. Haenszel W, Kurihara M. Studies of Japanese migrants. I. Mortality from cancer and other diseases among Japanese in the United States. J Natl Cancer Inst 1968; 40:43-68.

5. Shimizu H, Ross RK, Bernstein L, Yatani R, Henderson BE, Mack TM. Cancers of the prostate and breast among Japanese and white immigrants in Los Angeles County. Br J Cancer 1991; 63:963-966.

6. Hsing AW, Tsao L, Devesa SS. International trends and patterns of prostate cancer incidence and mortality. Int J Cancer 2000; 85:60-67.

7. Hemminki K, Lorenzo Bermejo J, Forsti A. The balance between heritable and environmental etiology of human disease. Nat Rev Genet. 2006 Dec; 7(12):958-65. PMID: 17139327

8. Hemminki. K, Forsti. A, Bermejo. JL, (2006). Gene-environment interactions in cancer: do they exist? Ann. N. Y. Acad. Sci. 1076: 137-148

9. Paul J (2006). 'Surveillance and management of all types of Staphylococcus aureus bacteraemia: MRSA policies divert attention from MSSA and may risk lives'. Brit Med J 333 (7562): 269-70.

10. Available at: http://www.cato.org/pubs/tbb/tbb_0925-40.pdf Accessed 2007-01-01

11. Acheson D. Independent inquiry into inequalities in health. London: Stationery Office, 1998(Acheson report.)

12. Black D, Morris JN, Smith C, Townsend P. Inequalities in health: report of a research working group. London: Department of Health and Social Security, 1980(Black report.)

13. Commission on Macroeconomics and Health. Macroeconomics and health: investing in health for economic development. Geneva: Commission on Macroeconomics and Health, 2001.

14. Suhrcke M, McKee M, Sauto Arce R, Tsolova S, Mortensen J. The contribution of health to the economy in the European Union. Brussels: European Commission, 2005.

15. Arora S. Health, human productivity, and long-term economic growth. J Econ Hist 2001; 61(3).

16. Sala-I-Martin X, Doppelhofer G, Miller RI. Determinants of long-term growth: a bayesian averaging of classical estimates (BACE) approach. Am Econ Rev 2004; 94:813-35.

17. Suhrcke M, Urban D. Is cardiovascular disease bad for economic growth? Venice: WHO European Office for Investment for Health and Development, 2006.

18. Theil, Henri (1964). Optimal Decision Rules for Government and Industry. Amsterdam: North Holland.

19. Tinbergen, Jan (1956). Economic Policy: Principles and Design. Amsterdam: North Holland.

20. The 2006-07 Infoway Corporate Business Plan. Available at: http://www.infoway-inforoute.ca/en/WorkingWithInfoway/PositionDescription.aspx?UID=109 Accessed on January 3, 2007

21. Schoen. C, Osborn. R, Trang Huynh. R, Doty. M, Peugh. J, and Kinga Zapert. On The Front Lines Of Care: Primary Care Doctors' Office Systems, Experiences, And Views In Seven Countries Health Affairs, 25, no. 6 (2006): w555-w571 doi: 10.1377/hlthaff.25.w555 Available at: http://content.healthaffairs.org/cgi/content/abstract/hlthaff.25.w555?ijkey=3YyH7yDwrJSoc&keytype=ref&siteid=healthaff Accessed on January 03, 2007

22. Available at: http://news.bbc.co.uk/2/hi/business/6227575.stm Accessed on January 3, 2007

23. Available at: http://news.bbc.co.uk/2/hi/technology/6224183.stm Accessed on January 3, 2007

24. Cutler. D, Deaton. A, Lleras-Muney. A. The Determinants of Mortality, *Journal of Economic Perspectives*, Vol 20, Number 3, Summer 2006.

25. Rogers, Richard G., Robert A. Hummer, and Charles B. Nam, *Living and dying in the USA. Behavioral, health, and social differences in adult mortality*, New York. Academic Press, 2000

26. Elo, Irma T. and Samuel H. Preston, "Educational Differentials in Mortality: United States, 1979-85," *Social Science and Medicine* 42(1), 1996

27. Costa, Dora L., and Richard H. Steckel, "Long Term Trends in Health, Welfare, and Economic Growth", in Richard H. Steckel and Robert Floud, eds., *Health and Welfare During Industrialization*, Chicago: University of Chicago Press, 1997.

28. Murphy, Kevin M. and Robert H. Topel, "The value of health and longevity," Cambridge, MA. NBER Working Paper No. 11045, June 2005.

29. Rogot, Eugene, Paul D. Sorlie, Norman J. Johnson, and Catherine Schmitt, *A Mortality Study of 1.3 million persons*, Bethesda, MD. National Institutes of Health, National Heart Lung, and Blood Institute, 1992.

30. Office of National Statistics, United Kingdom, 2005, "Trends in life-expectancy by social class 1972-2001",
http://www.statistics.gov.uk/downloads/theme_population/Life_Expect_Social_class_1972_01/Life_Expect_Social_Class_1972-2001.pdf
Accessed January 4, 2007

31. Available at:
http://www.nytimes.com/2007/01/03/health/03aging.html?_r=2&oref=slogin&ref=todayspaper&pagewanted=print&oref=slogin Accessed on January 4, 2007

The Future
Of
Private Health Insurance

Healthcare financing is changing, and inevitably so. The rapid emergence of new medical knowledge is spawning healthcare delivery paradigms, which along with progress in technology, generate increasingly critical analyses of the nature and extent of government involvement in healthcare financing, and of market failures. These developments raise important questions regarding not just the potency or otherwise of government in the new healthcare delivery dispensation, but also the implications for it, and for performance, and quality, of competition, ownership, and regulatory activities, among others. They also constitute the underlying currents for the evolution of private health insurance (PHI) in many countries, including those with predominantly publicly funded health systems. Indeed, governments frequently resort to private health insurance (PHI) in solving certain problems that their health systems face. They bolster PHI as an option in health financing, to augment system capacity, as a major healthcare coverage model, or even part of the framework for the achievement of their overall policy objectives, in the process oiling the machinery of the evolution of PHI, without necessarily shepherding the direction in which it transitions. Nonetheless, among the most important variables in the changes that PHI would undergo in the years ahead would be the continuing increase in health spending in many countries. Among countries in the Organization for Economic Cooperation and Development (OECD), for example, the persistence of this increase would likely result in governments increasing taxes, reducing spending in other sectors, or in more individual out-of-pocket health expenses, according to recent OECD data[1]. These data indicate that from 1990 to 2004, health spending increased more rapidly than Gross Domestic Product (GDP), 7% and 8.9% of GDP respectively, in all OECD countries but Finland. With these percentages expected to increase even further due to population aging and pricey medical technologies, the need for sustainable healthcare financing could not be direr in these countries, including Canada. Considering that most OECD countries finance health via taxes, in 2004, 73% of health spending averagely publicly funded the potential implications for the evolution of PHI, at once notional yet potentially critical, and by extension although not least also, those for the underlying fabric of healthcare delivery in tandem with its symbiotic dyadic with other sectors, on the overall economy. This is more so with more questions emerging regarding government's role in health services provision, with increasing service devolution to the private sector in some countries, the increasing role out-of-pocket private payments for health services in others, and in yet others, national, geopolitical and global economic realities, and the ever-changing key health sector payer-payee dynamics, among others, at play. These developments no doubt partly explain the decline, significant reversals in fact, in the public share of health spending in countries such as Hungary, the Czech Republic, and Poland, all May 01, 2004 entrants into the European Union (EU), among the last group of entrants before the latest, Romania and Bulgaria on January 01, 2007. On the other hand, countries such as Mexico, Korea, Switzerland, and the U.S., are using more tax money to fund their health systems[1], in the U.S., 40% to 45% from 1990 to 2004, public spending on health per capita more than in most OECD countries, as it spends more on health overall. Even then, in the U.S., the private sector still funds more health services than do taxes. The extent to which private payments for health, that is, those that PHI funds, and those paid for with out-of-pocket funds, contribute to healthcare financing is in general less in countries that operate publicly funded health systems, but for how long would this remain so? Mexico, Greece, and Korea, had the highest out-of-pocket spending among OECD countries in 2004, 51%, 45%, and 37%, respectively[1], PHI only about 6% averagely among OECD countries, 37% in the U.S., and 10% to 15 % in Canada and France, in the same year. The question though is whether, considering developments in the health and non-health domains, these figures would increase down the road. Private payments for health services seem to play a much larger role in funding medications, for example, than hospital or ambulatory services, as many publicly funded health insurance fund drugs inadequately, public spending in 2004 on drugs among OECD countries least in Mexico, U.S., Poland, and Canada, 12%, 24%, 37%, and 38%, respectively[1], versus over 70% in Austria and France. Would more Canadians for example need more medications, as the population ages, and the prevalence of chronic non-communicable diseases increases, or would there be a push toward the use of the cheaper, generics, in preference to the more expensive brand medications? Would issues such as efficacy, and even costs modulation that could make brand medications less expensive obviate this push, and what effects could these developments have on enrollment or otherwise in PHI schemes? PHI no doubt affects different health jurisdictions differently, presenting prospects and problems whose outcomes are equally contextual with regard the achievement by respective jurisdictions of their healthcare delivery objectives. Thus, in some countries, PHI helped infuse resources into health systems, making them more robust, and pliable, offering the healthcare consumer more options. In others, by increasing premium costs, it made them less affordable for many, creating inequities in healthcare delivery, which potentially could further compromise the health system, and the overall health of a country. Yet, in particular regarding this latter, the challenges posed by PHI reflect in the main the market failures mentioned earlier. It is uncertain the role that government plays in creating such situations, hence the rationality or otherwise of its intervention in for example modulating the contending forces of ensuring healthcare access simultaneously maintaining the vigorous and varied insurance coverage crucial to the efficient market operations that we seek. This situation is even more relevant to considerations of the role each objective plays in the sustenance of the other, and in that of the wider economic system, in a symbiotic dyadic, whose outcome feeds, in a systemic intercalation, into mutually constructive or destructive situations, a perpetual motion toward progress or decadence, ensuing, although tractable, even if not invariably so. In other words, we are in control of the processes that move the evolution of both the healthcare and its coverage in whatever direction, at least, in the main, even if some of the actions we need to take to ensure that neither is moribund, could be distressingly cryptic. In this regard, we must first acknowledge that the objectives of each do not necessarily have to collide, the sort of angst whose contemplation results in the adversarial hue critics of some health systems, such as that of the U.S., paint of their operators. We should then, in a systematic analysis of the issues involved explore the potential for collaboration among the drivers of each, within the context of the fundamental principles that assure the positive as opposed to the negative motion of both. This highlights the need to focus on the implications for contemporary healthcare delivery, the inherent tension between of the age-old transcendental versus positivist debate whose evolution as some would argue, nullifies itself for example, in the dissolution of the distinctions in Donald Davidson (1917-2003) and his teacher, W.V.O. Quine (1908-2000), between the semantic-pragmatic, the analytic-synthetic, the scheme-reality, and the linguistic-empirical. Yet, far from eschewing the need for us to commit to exploring healthcare delivery issues via methodological analysis and logical rigor, we, in acknowledging the evolution past 'classical logical positivism' of the healthcare delivery zeitgeist, also do, that of the continuing dialectic, process cycle analysis, fundamental to what should be our quest to achieve the dual healthcare delivery objectives (DHDO). These objectives, namely to provide qualitative health services efficiently and cost-effectively, would emerge in the continuous process that such analyses would spawn, a decomposition/exposition of key healthcare delivery issues, the determination of the modifiers/facilitators of which, would in addition to enabling progress, impel ongoing quality evaluation and control. This relieves the torment of the genuineness of agency and therefore of moral judgment with which many probably would agree in the argument for and against how much if any control we really have contrary to our earlier assertion, over the factors driving the issues in question. This makes the pursuance of the dual objectives mentioned above for example, an imperative for which we should morally account. This is so, among other reasons, considering their ramifications for our right to life, and the very survival of our countries, and indeed, our world, a Humean pragmatism to which few probably would object in keeping with the motion, in the main, of the individual/collective dyadic, toward life as opposed to death. Thus, we see the coalescence of the aversion to decadence to which we must all subscribe, one that neither the Platonist nor the positivist would eschew, one which as an underlying stratagem forges us in the direction of more perfection, in our healthcare delivery efforts, and indeed, in all else we do. In other words, we would recognize the need for us to pay attention to our health services, digging deep into the fundamental fabric of our lives, even if nothing else compels us so to do. Past merely the focus though, would be the realization of the need to ensure their continuous improvement, which indeed, the exigencies of our realities would increasingly demand.

The role that PHI would play in our efforts in this direction would likely be profound in the years ahead in many countries, or would it? Even in countries such as the U.S., where there is a significant complement of private health insurance, health financing with public funds is just as substantial. Given the aforementioned, our key goal is to achieve the provision of qualitative health services to all efficiently and cost-effectively. The question is how well the government is doing that, and if not so well, how much involvement of the private sector we need to spruce things up. Even in countries that predominantly fund their health services with tax revenues, there has been in recent times, an increasing private sector involvement in healthcare delivery. In the U.K., for example, PHI supplements the publicly funded National Health Service (NHS), whose 2006/7 budget is £96billion[2,] although the latter is 'free at the point of delivery.' With its annual deficit estimated to be almost £7bn in 2010[3], many would no doubt query how well the services run, and if the private sector should not in fact participate more in health services provision in the country. That publicly funded cognitive-behavioral therapy (CBT) for psychiatric disorders is scarce in Canada in spite of proven efficacy and guidelines recommending its use, is another case in point. A review of published data on the economic effects of CBT in the treatment of mental disorders for examples mood, anxiety, psychotic, and somatoform disorders, found that regardless of health care settings and patient populations, CBT alone or along with medications is offers satisfactory value for expended health dollars, less health services utilizing offsetting CBT costs[4]. The authors concluded that international evidence indicates that CBT is cost-effective, and that improved access to these services would likely improve outcomes and save costs. This would no doubt have some wondering if the effectiveness of efforts by the public health system to achieve the dual healthcare delivery objectives (DHDO), and if indeed, the private sector should not actively participate in providing such services and what this implies for PHI utilization down the road. Should we not in fact take this issue seriously, considering the potential value of CBT in reducing the burden, in human and material terms, of relatively common disorders such as depression? Ever since research evidence showed in the late 1980s and early 1990s that depression predicts outcome in patients recovering from heart attacks[5], interests in improving depression symptoms in patients with heart diseases enough with treatment to affect either the disease process or patient compliance thereby saving lives have continued unabated. Even if the effect on cardiac outcomes of treating depression were likely a function of this exercise as it were of its effect on the processes in the heart's functioning connecting depression with outcome, could we not be achieving much knowing for example, the specific interventions for depression that could reduce the incidence of cardiac events, say, heart attacks? The desirability of being able to do so is hardly in doubt, but should we not consider the implications thereof, increasing the prevalence of heart failure, for instance, and should we not also want to do something about it? Whereas the prevalence of cardiovascular disease is generally declining in developed countries, heart failure is ironically, becoming more prevalent due to improved survival of patients with cardiovascular disease and population aging[6, 7]. Furthermore, heart failure has with very high morbidity and mortality rates, the cause of more than 106,000 hospital admissions and 1,400,000 inpatient days in Canada in 2000[8], and coronary artery disease (CHD) is the single most important cause, indeed the primary cause in over 70%, of all heart failure cases[9], coronary ischemia, not controlled, a common cause of heart-failure flare-ups[10]. Should we therefore not follow the recommendations in practice guidelines for patients with heart failure and CHD to have coronary revascularization[9], for examples coronary-artery bypass grafting (CABG) or percutaneous coronary intervention (PCI), support for the benefits of which there is research evidence[8, 11]? There is little doubt about these issues gaining increasing prominence in developed countries in future, with significant implications for the roles of public vis-à-vis private insurance, because of the costs of routine revascularization in an increasing number of patients not to mention the 'wait times' issues this would likely spawn, among other related but important issues that could arise. Does it have implications for cost sharing also considering the fact that the prevailing model for demand-side cost sharing for example trades off moral hazard in relation to risk evasion? If so what effect could the chances that lower cost sharing for some medications, and indeed, other treatment and services, could reduce overall health care costs eventually, have on the potential for the widespread adoption of this model and for PHI even in countries with predominantly publicly funded health systems? Could the increased use of certain services with lower costs sharing that eventually reduces overall healthcare costs, and hence spending, by improving overall health including those of individuals with self-discipline problems actually mean cost sharing could be applicable in publicly funded health systems? Does it also mean that it makes sense for employers in the private sector to offer health financial support, which would eventually improve their firms' productivity and reduce labor costs, rather than exclude potentially valuable services screening workers and applicants for say, obesity, or cigarette smoking? Are these issues not also pertinent for society as whole with the call by some for example to legislate public health and indeed, the passage of bylaws in many health jurisdictions, banning the cigarette smoking in public places? In other words, should these jurisdictions be asking smokers to pay part of the costs of the treatments of their smoking-related health conditions, smoking in designated bars, for example, while still banning smoking in public places to prevent non-smokers developing health issues related to passive smoking? What are the implications for PHI for example, of the decision in November 2005 by three Suffolk, U.K., primary care trusts not to provide operations such as hip and knee replacement surgeries, to patients with a body mass index (BMI) over 30, classed as obese, which roughly 40% of doctors in the British Medical Association (BMA) News survey supported[12]. About the same percentage of the doctors also supported barring smokers and drinkers from certain procedures the bans, however, on medical, rather than costs grounds. These issues point to the likelihood that even publicly funded health systems such as in the U.K., would over time come to rely increasingly more of the private sector for service provision, as the public system increasingly becomes unable to cope for a variety of reasons providing the quality levels of care that an increasingly enlightened and suave public demands. Could such publicly funded systems avoid this fate, and is it in fact necessary that they attempt to do so? What does a recent leaked U.K. government document indicating that there would be a dearth of GPs and nurses in four years although the NHS will have to reduce the number of doctors[13], and indeed, carry out wide-ranging job cuts, about 2.7%, or 37,000 jobs in 2007 alone, to save funds. The leaked Department of Health document, piece of the draft of the 2008/2022 NHS pay and workforce strategy, showed that there would be a shortfall of 1,200 GPs, 14,000 nurses, and 1,100 junior and stag grade doctors by 2011. Further, the NHS would not be able to pay 3,200 additional consultants and 16,000 other health professionals for examples, physiotherapists, health scientists, and technicians. What do the measures suggested in the draft document such as nurses' salary dictated by local market rates, utilizing unemployment to 'create downward pressure on wages,' creating a new grade of sub-consultants, and the use of temporary staff and short-term contracts, for the future of the NHS vis-à-vis private sector participation in health services delivery? Would these measures not compound the 'wait times' issue in the country and compromise health services delivery to the many, particularly, the elderly, the unemployed, and retirees, who might not be able to afford PHI, or would the operations of market forces result in some sort of 'down-regulation' of the costs of premiums, in keeping with the trade-off mentioned earlier? What knock-on effect could this have on workload pressure of retained staff, and their morale, even health, and efficiency, and what effect would this have on the quality of the health services delivered, on patients, and the overall health of the country, and by extension on its economic productivity? Do other publicly funded health systems such as Canada face similar problems down the road, and how could they avert such developments, if indeed, they should? The example of the U.K., raises certain fundamental issues germane to not just the British citizen, but to the health system, and indeed, to the country, and these issues apply not just to the U.K., but also to all other countries. In the first place, it raises the question of the commitment to the provision of health services to all that we all share, a commitment rooted in the need for the preservation of the basic right of each person to life. This right coalesces in reciprocity between the elements resultant, in that of the community in tandem with that of the individual to life, and by extension in that of the country to survive let alone thrive. Furthermore, there is evidence to support the tendency for health to affect a country's economy positively or otherwise directly, its overall health if poor, adversely affecting its productivity, hence its economy, not to mention the potentially massive drain on which latter the burden of disease could cause[14,15,16].

Given the above facts that any country could afford not to attempt to provide qualitative health services to its peoples, cost-effectively and efficiently seems, counterintuitive. This buttresses the point made earlier regarding the need for all health jurisdictions to pursue the achievement of the dual healthcare delivery objectives (DHDO), including investments in the appropriate healthcare information and communication technologies (healthcare ICT) that research evidence indicates could help in so doing. An example is a RAND Corporation study published in the journal *Health Affairs* on September 14, 2005, which noted that America's healthcare system could save over US$81 billion annually and improve the quality of care were it to widely adopt electronic medical records[17]. According to Richard Hillestad, a RAND senior management scientist who led the two-year study, the health system would save US$77 billion annually resulting from improved efficiencies if 90% of doctors and hospitals successfully adopted healthcare ICT. He noted that most savings would be from reduced hospital stays due to enhanced care coordination; streamlined workflow for example less nursing time expended on administrative tasks; more rational and safer medication use in hospitals; and of drugs, labs and radiology services in outpatient sites. Improved safety, essentially via reduced prescription errors with computerized alert systems warning doctors and pharmacists of would-be errors would save an extra US$4 billion annually[17]. Clearly, even an upfront investment in these technologies albeit the benefits not immediately evident would be prudent, which as evidence shows that in the same country, and indeed, in others such as Canada, the widespread adoption and utilization of these technologies still appears not so imminent[18], suggests the need for additional efforts in this direction, in these countries. This issue becomes even more relevant considering the increasing health spending in these and other developed countries, and the potential for these expenditures to increase further due to population aging. Because there is of necessity scarcity, since we cannot provide for all the wants of everyone all the time that we would need to optimize the allocation and use of these scarce resources is inevitable. These necessities also imply that the private health insurance sector, as noted earlier, would likely play an increasingly role in healthcare delivery in many countries, including those with mainly publicly funded health systems such as the U.K, and Canada, although the path toward this increased role would largely be contextual. This does not mean that the context in particular countries would necessarily be benign platforms on which private health insurance gleefully glide. Indeed, the evolution of health insurance along this path would be on the other hand likely bumpy, as the tussle with public health insurance would continue, and indeed, intensify as governments struggle to fulfill their mandates to the people. The example of California's Gov. Arnold Schwarzenegger, who proposed on January 8, 2007 to extend health coverage to almost all of the state's 6.5 million uninsured people, with a pledge to dissipate the cost among firms, individuals, hospitals, physicians, insurers and government, illustrates this point[19]. The Governor's plan underscores the position about the direction of motion of healthcare service provision being properly the preservation of the right of individuals to life, which guarantees that of society to survive and prosper. As if to demonstrate that this fact, rooted in the fundamental processes on which our world depends for its very survival, has everything for everyone, the Governor included in it, inducements for the miscellaneous interests groups expected to oppose the plan, which among others, guarantees healthcare coverage for all children, their immigration status regardless. This would be via an extension of the state and federal Healthy Families program. According to Gov. Arnold Schwarzenegger, 'I don't think it is a question or a debate if they ought to be covered. ... The federal courts have made that decision — that no one can be turned away....The question really isn't to treat them or not to treat them. The question really is how you can treat them in the most cost-effective way.' This is the key point, one that assumes the provision of qualitative and efficient services in short that hinges his plan, everyone having health insurance, the financially challenged, an estimated 1.2 million of them, subsidized, essentially on the achievement of the dual healthcare delivery objectives. According to the plan, firms that have over 10 employees would provide them health coverage or pay 4% of their payroll into a state fund, those with fewer employees, excused, insurers barred from denying persons coverage due to their medical conditions, the poor able to purchase coverage via a state-run pool and contribute a little something toward their premiums. Does the tradeoff between moral hazard vis-à-vis risk evasion, mentioned earlier not ring true here, and is it unconscionable the role that cost sharing would play in this and our future formulations to ensure the resolution of the competition-collaboration conundrum inherent in the interplay of forces crucial to our very existence? Would the extent to which the latter would feature in particular formulations not likely determine that to which in it PHI would also feature? The Governor estimates that the plan would save $10 billion per annum, slashing health care costs, savings he envisages would offset the new fees doctors and hospitals would pay, 4% and 2% of revenue for hospitals and doctors, respectively, albeit the state increasing coverage payments for the underprivileged to both, via Medi-Cal. Again, this illustrates the new look of the complicated formulations that health jurisdictions would increasingly need to develop to achieve the dual healthcare delivery objectives. It is also an indication of the dichotomy in roles between government and other healthcare stakeholders that would be equally indispensable to the achievement of these goals, the challenges posed thereof, which we would not only have to confront but to necessarily overcome. The differences in position between that of the Democrats and the Republicans in the U.S., on the 2003 Medicare law prohibiting direct negotiations by government with drug companies, preferring private insurance firms and their agents, to secure reduced drug prices for Medicare recipients that the former want to repeal, is instructive in this regard[20]. This is so in particular regarding, as the Health and Human Services Secretary Michael Leavitt noted, if the government's recent announcement of a 10% reduction in the last six months in the costs estimates of Medicare's new prescription drug benefit indicate the efficient operations of market forces. In effect, that competition among private plans resulted in prices falling, and that government's interference in these negotiations would result in less choices and compromise consumer satisfaction, and by extension that this interference could stymie the fall in prices, which would work against the interests of seniors who the Democrats argue are still paying too much for these drugs. That the estimated payments for private plans in July 2006 for Medicare services provision from 2007-2016, was $1.077 trillion, and now $964 billion is also instructive vis-à-vis the future of PHI in the country, in particular enrollment in the new Medicare program is lower than anticipated, some recipients realizing they had comparable medication coverage elsewhere. Here then is the potential origin of the competition that could emerge between the public and the private health sectors. In a country such as Canada, this would of course play out slightly differently but the underlying drivers would be similar. With the increasing renewed, interest in the New Public Management (NPM) principles, the critical reform measures implied in which many governments have seemingly, some would argue, paid lip service, that we would more likely see this competition play out in many countries, including Canada, is near certainty. There is no doubt that every public service sector needs to be more efficient, and the likelier this would be the more market-oriented its management is. So, would we need and inevitably so, to embrace more forcefully, in the public health sector, NPM principles? The answer is affirmative, more so considering the increasing need for more efficiency and cost-effectiveness in the health, and indeed, other sectors of our economy. In June 2006, the OECD released its annual Employment Outlook and a supplementary report, *Boosting Jobs and Incomes*, in which it urged OECD countries to get more people into paid employment urgently, if they wanted to boost living standards and keep welfare systems going[21]. It further advised them to eschew policies that discourage people from working and firms from hiring and focus more on improving workers' skills. It noted that many individuals on welfare see minimal financial gain in taking up employment, and those that want to or do, hindered by adverse regulations, deficient job-search support, or inadequate skill sets, the combination in turn hampering economic growth and prosperity. If we accepted the recommendations in these two reports, which essentially comprise the outcome of a two-year evaluation of employment policies in the OECD, and how effective its Jobs Strategy launched in 1994 is, we would need to emphasize, not just macroeconomic stability via policies aimed at achieving price stability, and sustainable public finances, but also a solid market orientation[21]. The implications of these measures for health reform are undoubted, considering population aging, for example, with more seniors in jobs, hence more likely to be able to afford PHI when for example, they perceived the public system having failed them. Would this mean easing the restriction on the services purchasable from the private sector that Medicare also covers, in for example, to prevent capital flight, these seniors seeking these services outside the country, venturing out of Quebec, for example? How much easing would this mean and what could be the consequences for the economic viability of the public health system, in that particular jurisdiction, which did not provide satisfactory services, in terms of loss of patronage? Could this result in the evolution of a parallel private health sector in the country, and is this evolution inevitable, and what would this mean for the widespread use of PHI? This example also illustrates the point made earlier regarding the need for us to rededicate ourselves to NPM principles, with the public health services, as with core private sector business principles, adopting a more efficiency-oriented approach to the conduct of their affairs, as opposed to ideological-based political expediency, often predicated on public opinion itself based on inadequate information. This information asymmetry incidentally pervades the health sector, its roots, at least partly, in the atavistic paternalism the medical profession struggles to shake off, realizing, as it should, the need for patients to be fully aware of health information that would help them in making discerning judgments on matters pertaining to their health and to health in general. Part of our reform process in the health sector, would therefore involve making information available, and ensuring that it reaches those that need it, an exercise that the widespread adoption and implementation of healthcare information and communication technologies would facilitate in achieving. The upfront investments in these technologies therefore, coupled with other necessary measures that would boost employment would be worthwhile considering the warning by OECD for example that countries that do not reform would likely experience persistent weak employment performance with the potential to compromise living standards, and by extension health. This would increase the burden of disease, in human and material times, costing us even more eventually.

Another recent OECD publication, Economic Survey of Canada 2006: Managing the challenges ahead[22], noted the excellent performance of the country's economy, with even the economies of the slowest-growing provinces/territories, still expanding at about 2% per annum. However, it also noted that major challenges are ahead, for example, the potential adverse effects of rapid population ageing vis-à-vis workforce size, which could compromise public finances via an increase in elderly and health care spending, which that our hourly productivity growth in the business sector has been feeble lately, albeit it increased in 2005, does not seem to help. Therefore, we need to improve productivity performance to ensure that long-term prosperity accrues, which our current high employment rates, would facilitate, even if we also needed to ensure that we have sustainable fiscal social welfare policies, the cost of shifting from welfare to work by modifying policies on benefits loss, including health coverage and housing, which we do. The relationship between health and the economy is not in doubt, is essential bidirectional, although the influence of the former on the latter seems more dramatic. Nonetheless, it is doubtful that an ever-increasing health bill for the country would be sustainable in the long term. Yet, as with many other OECD countries, health spending in Canada keeps rising, which as earlier mentioned, the OECD noted if persistent, would result in tax increases, reduced expenditure on other services, even increased out-of-pocket health expenditure[1]. We would need to avoid these consequences, among others would likely need avoided by even the most skeptics of the potential benefits of ongoing health reform, including emphasis on the promotion of the widespread adoption and utilization of healthcare information and communications technologies in healthcare delivery in the country. It is the very combination of the consequences of such widespread adoption on the healthcare consumer, and the provider, that would drive the future of healthcare delivery in the country, specifically, that regarding the adoption or otherwise of a parallel private health system and its nature and extent. Unlike the formulations, though that puts the public health system at a loss because of this evolution, the interplay of a variety of other factors would contrariwise position the public health system positively, to compete favorably among sundry health systems, including those in the public sector. Thus, what we would see is competition among public health systems, between public and private health systems, and between private and private health systems. The interplay of a variety of forces, both within and outside the health system would therefore, result in a comprehensive competitive, albeit collaborative, milieu, which would result in a more perfect overall health system in the country. The fundamental basis of this scenario would be the ascendancy of the healthcare consumer over time. The result of our efforts to redress the information asymmetry mentioned above would be profound, as the Canadian healthcare consumer becomes equipped more and more with the tools to make discerning decisions. These smarter choices would have implications for health and healthcare, preventive and curative, with implications also for society's overall health, and as we noted earlier, in turn that of the country's economy. It is difficult to see how anyone would contend paying attention to the mechanisms that result in such desirable results, and the desirability is not whimsical, borne of deep-seated philosophical roots, attention to which is inevitable considering the preferred tendency to the right to life discussed earlier than to death. Here again, we see the central role that healthcare ICT would play in the entire process, starting with rectifying information asymmetry. Additionally, these technologies would help reduce transaction costs, which constitute a significant percentage of the Gross National Product (GNP) in developed countries such as Canada[23], one reason, among others that the public services in Canada need to re-embrace so to say, the New Public Management (NPM) principles mentioned earlier. That government should transition from 'a concern to do, towards a concern to ensure that things are done,' as Kaul noted[24], the fundamental platform of the NPM principle, is not in doubt. This is more so, as reducing the costs associated with exchange for example, and indeed, more complex hence higher costs, than in many other instances, the activities involved in healthcare delivery, would be likelier within market-based rather than hierarchical control processes. Furthermore, and in particular in our country, and many other developed countries, the institutional arrangements are in existence, and have garnered over time immense public trust, which could ensure the former operates efficiently and cost-effectively, further making the potential of such operations helping to reduce transaction costs likelier. These issues also highlight the importance of rectifying information asymmetry, which has close links with transaction costs, the exchange itself essentially a principal giving the responsibility for a task to an agent, in healthcare delivery, the healthcare consumer, and the doctor, for examples, respectively. In this particularly instance, equipping the healthcare consumer with the relevant information would doubtless, mitigate the risks, with some such agents, to allow their commitments to other principals, for example, the health authorities for which they work, to conflict with their contractual obligations to the healthcare consumer. Because of the potential assemblage of principal-agent relationships in healthcare delivery, this sort of 'confusion' or even 'conflict of interests' are almost invariable, although not solvable. Indeed, the well-informed healthcare consumer could shift patronage elsewhere, which speaks to the preference of market-type health systems, although a public health system that has embraced the NPM principles mentioned above would have 'embedded' in every aspect of the exchange, accountability checks that would also help reduce such conflicts. This latter speaks to the public health system, not necessarily becoming moribund with the emergence of the PHI, for example. Besides the healthcare consumer being able to exit a situation and the hierarchical assurance of accountability via the system, that the healthcare consumer, armed with the required information, is able to add his/her voice, in a democratic milieu toward influencing healthcare delivery, the three key mechanisms in ensuring accountability that Paul (1992) [25]noted, are instructive in this regard. No doubt, scale economies could reduce the potency of consumer choice, as it becomes harder for the healthcare consumer to access service quality, which underscores the need for the availability of adequate and current information on services to the healthcare consumer, were the concept of consumer choice to work, even in the public sector, where scale economies are often minimal. This is why, we cannot afford to ignore Paul's two other key mechanisms mentioned above, with for example having ombudsmen and establishing hospital committees to hear from the healthcare consumer and investigate his/her complaints, ensuring we include those of the vulnerable among us, the underprivileged, the disabled, and the frail, for examples. The increasing appreciation of the efficiency and cost-effectiveness of such horizontal approaches to ensuring accountability and fostering consumer choice, for examples, would be inevitable as we also appreciate the central figure of the healthcare consumer in the healthcare delivery process. This is, among others, because the care of the healthcare consumer after all, is the reason there are healthcare services in the first place. Furthermore, and in assuring the best quality service provision in delivering this care, we cannot afford to cripple other aspects of our social and economic well-being. In fact, these two and others, depend on the health and well-being of the individual healthcare consume, and in turn on that of the community. The intricacies of the interrelationships between these different entities and situations are to say the least intriguing. This is more so as we the tendency mentioned above to evolve in a direction that might not be very surprising, albeit not necessarily immediately obvious. This direction would involve, as our discussion so far shows, the increasing incursion of market operations in healthcare delivery. This would be so as the need to embrace the most efficient and cost-effective exchanges within buoyant regulatory milieus, just as efficient and cost-effect, ex ante, finding the most appropriate contractor and instituting the contract, and ex post, monitoring and regulating the contractor, for examples, becomes the norm. That government's role in health services provision would be less direct, and that of the healthcare consumer more intense would lead us in this direction predicates on the appreciation, in fact, for millennia, evident in the evolution of thought from the days of Plato's *The Republic*, of the links between the reasons we justify political authority and human nature. Thus, we have transitioned from the philosopher-king, to Aristotle's suggestion of an aristocracy of the able and virtuous wielding political power, in *The Nicomachean Ethics* and *The Politics*, which latter ideas, much later, Niccolò Machiavelli (1469 –1527), opposed, arguing that rather than signifying moral virtues, the sovereign conducts the necessary. Thomas Hobbes' (1588-1679) assertion that the sovereign by common agreement delivers us from the 'state of nature,' also received strong opposition in particular from Jean-Jacques Rousseau, whose 'noble-savage' view of human nature soiled if anything by social contract, John Locke (1632-1704), built on that the state of nature that could ensue with government intervention might be worse than the Hobbesian.

Thus, despite the term democracy emerging from Greece millennia before, its

elements started to emerge more fully in the body polity thenceforth, the evolution of private health insurance that we have thus described, an integral part of that of healthcare delivery within the overall system that we would be hard-pressed to find justification for stopping even if we could. This evolution would occur in fact in every corner of the globe, albeit at different rates, and over different periods. It is increasingly clear that as we redress information asymmetry, we have to respect the choices one another makes, as incidentally Hobbes also noted, the right to life prevails, and with blurring of the distinction between the Judeo-Christian and Hobbesian (reverse) Golden Rules, the need for a Leviathan to enforce the healthy competition/collaboration mix that would result, evidently unnecessary. The institutions necessary to advance the processes involved in the evolution in the direction mentioned would emerge in different societies due to this right to life prevailing, a right that obscures the evolution of the 'fact-value distinction' that some argue started with the skepticism of David Hume (1711-1776), and attenuated the arguments for political power derivable from nature. It is so because what is, the positive, or fact, is not always distinct, from what ought to be, the normative, value, or consensual. Indeed, unlike the Humean position that we cannot derive normative from positive arguments, or 'what ought' from 'is,' one could argue for the bidirectional relationship between these two forms of arguments. For example, that the values of scientists and the public have stymied the intentions of some scientists in the UK to breed a cow/human hybrid to study diseases and their cures, would influence the facts we know about those diseases is not in doubt. Similarly, the fact that we are first biological entities that must survive for us to develop values is indubitable, these two examples, indicative of the blurred distinction between the fact and value, rendering it redundant. Also similarly, the 'naturalistic fallacy', expounded by G.E. Moore (1873-1958), in the 'appeal to nature' form most used, which is different from the semantic/metaphysical fundamentals of ethics in which sense he described it in *Principia Ethica* (1903) is equally redundant. In other words, we are not here concerned with the goodness or otherwise of the evolutionary processes involved in healthcare delivery, but in their inevitability. We also not ascertaining the course of this evolution, as this would be essentially contextual, but its direction in which the evolution will proceed. We are asserting the coalescence of the 'ought to' and the 'is.' Thus that these processes are ongoing does not necessarily make them natural, as we have seen, and as we discussed earlier the bidirectional nature of the relationship between the 'ought to' and the 'is' suggests an evolutionary analytic. This, even receiver operating characteristics (ROC) curves in psychophysics for example remind us regarding the discriminating power of humans in detecting weak signals, which accords to scientific observations, potentially significant roles for the 'philosophic value,' of scientific enquiry, in shaping the facts of such enquiry. In other words, even the so-called, 'disruptive' events in science, and the polity, are unable to significantly, derail the ongoing exercises that we would necessarily conduct essentially in our efforts to achieve the right to life, via the achievement for example, regarding healthcare delivery that of the dual healthcare delivery objectives (DHDO). There are of course several options in addressing the imperfections inherent in the here and now such defective discriminatory capabilities spawn, but their paths are towards either life or death eventually, the aggregate likely towards the former, giving human actions. Otherwise, we would not have been able to survive in the wild with man-eating creatures multiple times our size all around us as we evidently did over the millennia. It is irrelevant if we called this process natural or not, it ought to or is, or indeed, good or bad. What matters is it is an ongoing process that will ensure our perpetual existence, our earth no longer does notwithstanding, provided of course we moved elsewhere prior. The idea then is that we need to start to examine our options regarding the public and private health care delivery mix that would ensure that we not just survive as a country but also thrive. As we have noted, the distinction between fact and value could sometimes not be so clear, and in fact need not be considering the close association between the two. This is why neither could be static or ignore developments in the other. The key issue in the end would be for each health jurisdiction to conduct its own and ongoing process cycle analysis, to determine, among others, the variety of issues and processes germane to health services delivery in its particular domain, and working with all healthcare stakeholders in one way or another, establish the most appropriate solutions to the issues. There are certain commonalities among processes though despite their differences, one being the crucial need to rectify information asymmetry in the healthcare delivery enterprise. This is a generic issue that no health jurisdiction could claim not to have, and indeed, is not solvable totally, as new information constantly emerges, nor, partly for this reason, some would argue indeed, desirable to commit inordinate efforts and resources so to do. Here again, the efforts that a particular health jurisdiction puts into rectifying this problem would vary with health jurisdiction. Another generic issue is the need to invest in and promote the acquisition and utilization by all healthcare stakeholders of healthcare information and communication technologies, again, the nature and extent of the efforts essentially contextual. It is within these contexts that PHI would evolve its nature, and pace contextual too. That not anticipating this evolution and making the necessary preparations and adjustments in our health services would likely have adverse consequences, not just for our health systems, but also our economy, that we neither need, not could not avoid. There is no doubt that we would need to strengthen current institutions and indeed, establish new ones to meet the challenges the ascendancy of PHI would have on not just Medicare, but also the overall health of Canadians, and the country's economy. This is because this ascendancy would not just involve internal health insurance in conjunction with a variety of models of private healthcare establishments and facilities, but competition between them and foreign investors in the country, on the one hand, and even with health facilities and insurers that do not even operate within Canada. These latter would include those for example, that have set up facilities in countries where it is cheaper to employ doctors, and other healthcare professionals, or those that offer outsourcing services. As our campaigns against smoking, overweight/obesity improve, with the healthcare consumer not only having information but those that could lead directly or indirectly to action towards healthier lifestyles, progress in consumer electronics and other technologies continue to offer products and services that make life more enjoyable and less boring, Canadians would live longer and healthier lives. This also means that the evolution of the healthcare system, including PHI described thus far would accelerate, with potential consequences for the country's economy that could wipe out the gains we have made hitherto, if we did not make these necessary preparations in anticipation of the future, and to be sure, we have no time to spare. There is no doubt that Canadians would be receptive to a comprehensive dialogue on issues pertaining to their health. It would even be much easier to engage the populace, the required information crucial to a fuller understanding of the intimate link between health and the economy, and the significant role that the adoption and utilization of healthcare information and communication technologies would play in ensuring that the overall health of Canadians continues to be high. It would therefore, be necessary to emphasize during the dialogue, which should have all the trappings of the workings of an efficient democracy, the need for us all to promote the health and well-being of not just ourselves and those close to us but also of all Canadians. This would ensure that the country's health sector has a positive effect on the economy. This exercise is crucial in tackling successfully, many of the country's healthcare delivery issues, including for example, that of hospital 'wait times.' For example, healthcare consumers would have a clearer understanding of the importance of healthcare ICT in solving this problem, and of simple measures that healthcare consumers could take, such as canceling appointments they would miss in advance, rather than simply not showing up, which also is important in so doing. There is no doubt that we would continue to improve healthcare delivery in the country, but we need to be aware of the 'wind of change' literally that is blowing across the country's healthcare delivery spectrum, paying attention to, and addressing the issues relevant to which, would make it much easier for us to achieve the DHDO. This would not only mean that we would continue to improve our health services, and enjoy even higher standards of care, but also of living in general, as the improved health system, also improves the economy, even if incrementally, and in the long term. The task of improving of health system is therefore not just that of the public health system, but would increasingly be that of all of us, including the private health sector, and increasing too, of private health insurance. We must do this task.

References

1. Available at: http://www.oecd.org/document/37/0,2340,en_2649_37407_36986213_1_1_1_37407,00.html Accessed on January 5, 2007

2. HM Treasury (2006-03-22). Budget 2006

3. YouGov (2006-03-09). NHS: How Well Is Our Money Being Spent?

4. Myhr G. Payne K. Cost-effectiveness of cognitive-behavioral therapy for mental disorders: implications for public health care funding policy in Canada. [Review] [52 refs] [Journal Article. Review] Canadian Journal of Psychiatry - Revue Canadienne de Psychiatrie. 51(10):662-70, 2006 Sep.

5. Frasure-Smith N, Lespérance F. Recent evidence linking coronary heart disease and depression. Can J Psychiatry 2006; 51:730 –7.

6. Tsuyuki RT, Shibata MC, Nilsson C, et al. Contemporary burden of illness of congestive heart failure in Canada. Can J Cardiol 2003; 19:436-8.

7. Liu P, Arnold M, Belenkie I, et al. The 2001 Canadian Cardiovascular Society consensus guideline update for the management and prevention of heart failure. Can J Cardiol 2001; 17(Suppl E):5E-24E.

8. Ross T. Tsuyuki, Fiona M. Shrive, P. Diane Galbraith, Merril L. Knudtson, Michelle M. Graham for the APPROACH Investigators Revascularization in patients with heart failure Can. Med. Assoc. J., Aug 2006; 175: 361 – 365

9. Hunt SA, Baker DW, Chin MH, et al. ACC/AHA guidelines for the evaluation and management of chronic heart failure in the adult: a report of the American College of Cardiology/American Heart Association Task Force on Practice Guidelines (Committee to Revise the 1995 Guidelines for the Evaluation and Management of Heart Failure. J Am Coll Cardiol 2001; 38:2101-13.

10. Opasich C, Febo O, Riccardi G, et al. Concomitant factors of decompensation in chronic heart failure. Am J Cardiol 1996; 78:354-7.

11. Baker DW, Jones R, Hodges J, et al. Management of heart failure. III. The role of revascularization in the treatment of patients with moderate or severe left ventricular systolic dysfunction. JAMA 1994; 272:1528-34.

12. Available at: http://news.bbc.co.uk/2/hi/health/4674594.stm Accessed on January 7, 2007

13. Available at: http://news.bbc.co.uk/2/hi/health/6228659.stm Accessed on January 7, 2007

14. Commission on Macroeconomics and Health. Macroeconomics and health: investing in health for economic development. Geneva: Commission on Macroeconomics and Health, 2001.

15. Suhrcke M, McKee M, Sauto Arce R, Tsolova S, Mortensen J. The contribution of health to the economy in the European Union. Brussels: European Commission, 2005.

16. Arora S. Health, human productivity, and long-term economic growth. J Econ Hist 2001; 61(3).

17. Available at: http://www.rand.org/news/press.05/09.14.html Accessed on January 7, 2007

18. Schoen. C, Osborn. R, Trang Huynh. R, Doty. M, Peugh. J and Kinga Zapert. On The Front Lines Of Care: Primary Care Doctors' Office Systems, Experiences, And Views In Seven Countries Health Affairs, 25, no. 6 (2006): w555-w571 doi: 10.1377/hlthaff.25.w555 Available at: http://content.healthaffairs.org/cgi/content/abstract/hlthaff.25.w555?ijkey=3YyH7yDwrJSoc&keytype=ref&siteid=healthaff Accessed on January 03, 2007

19. Available at: http://news.yahoo.com/s/ap/20070108/ap_on_re_us/california_health_care&printer=1 Accessed on January 8, 2007

20. Available at: http://www.nytimes.com/2007/01/07/washington/07medicare.html?_r=2&adxnnl=0&oref=slogin&adxnnlx=1168290229-uN9xl7JdguXx0ygy6qDpWA&pagewanted=print Accessed on January 8, 2007

21. Available at: http://www.oecd.org/document/31/0,2340,en_2649_201185_36899679_1_1_1_1,00.html Accessed on January 11, 2007

22. Available at: http://www.oecd.org/document/16/0,2340,en_2649_201185_36951632_1_1_1_1,00.html Accessed on January 11, 2007

23. North, D.C (1990) Institutions, Institutional Change, and Economic Performance. Cambridge University press, Cambridge.

24. Kaul, M (1997) The New Public Administration: management innovation in government. Public Administration and Development. 17:13-26

25. Paul, S. Accountability in public services: exit, voice, and control. World Development 20 (7): 1047-60.

On An Appeal to Nature

That health spending is increasing faster than incomes in most industrialized countries raises questions regarding its sustainability and future healthcare financing, particularly in countries such as the United States, which not just spends considerably more per capita on health care than any other country, but the rates of whose health spending also increase fastest[1], among developed countries. Indeed, health care spending is increasing faster than overall economic growth globally, its proportion of the gross domestic product (GDP), inflation-adjusted, increasing in virtually all countries, in the U.S., for example, from 8.8% in 1980 to 15.2% in 2003, 7.1% to 9.9% in Canada, and 5.6% to 7.8% in the U.K., over the same period[1]. The per capita health expenditures for 2003 in U.S. dollars purchasing power parity in the U.S., Canada, and the U.K., respectively, were $5,711, $2,998, and $ 2,317, and in Australia, and Sweden, $2,886, and $2,745, respectively. The two questions raised earlier become more pertinent considering that increased health spending does not necessarily correspond to improved health services or health indicators[2]. This no doubt calls for concerns, and justifiably so, regarding what policy makers, and indeed, all healthcare stakeholders could do to ensure that health systems provide value for the increasing health spending. Estimating the value of our health services, their relative effectiveness, or significance as judged by specific qualities, is indeed, central to any effort to improve their worth, to which decomposing the conceptual challenges we face concerning the issue of measuring the quality of healthcare delivery is therefore, germane. It is also important to consider the dimensions of health care performance, for examples access, cost, efficiency, and equity, and those of non-heath related factors such as system design, policy, and context. Categorization schemes for healthcare quality indicators abound. Donabedian for example described these indicators as being structure, process, or outcome in nature[4]. Structural indicators, or input indicators such as hospitals being well equipped, and the availability and suitability of healthcare professionals, no doubt could significantly boost or compromise health services provision. These factors are necessary but on their own cannot guarantee qualitative health services delivery, for example, that processes are appropriate, efficient and cost-effective, or that outcomes are satisfactory. The relevance of process indicators for example, if women had pap smears as appropriate predicates on healthcare delivery to at-risk populations being based on clinical evidence of the effectiveness of the process concerned and 'consistent with current knowledge'[5]. Thus, experts consider that they most closely reflect healthcare quality, than structural, or outcome indicators, the latter, for example, rates of nosocomial infections, which reflect improvements or otherwise consequent upon service provision, which other factors outside care quality, for example with nosocomial or hospital-acquired infections, an individual's immune status, could influence. Yet, we want to ensure that our measure of the quality of care contributes independently to it, hence the need to control, by risk adjustment for example, for other factors that influence healthcare delivery outcomes. This scheme no doubt has practical implications, which however, would remain heuristics, an iterative complexity that could only compromise our quality improvement efforts, if we lacked a comprehensive knowledge and appreciation of the fundamental issues and processes that would enable us determine the most appropriate interventions to improve these healthcare quality indicators. This presumes that some of these issues and processes would be peculiar to particular health jurisdictions, which makes the need to understand the local flavor that imbues them even more imperative. It also would reveal in the variety of symbiotic dyadic, health, and non-health, within and between jurisdictions, evident with such understanding, the fundamental motion of health systems, which determine the direction of their evolution. That this motion accelerates or decelerates, or indeed, wobbles on a spot, which among others the healthcare quality indicators would show, would be equally evident of the nature of our current interventions and the extent or otherwise to which they influence the direction in which our health services head. The transition from the situation we are in regarding our health systems, and the positive indicators we seek could be chiasmic, given the potential for us to ground the normative in the positive, the very Humean antithesis that we, nonetheless, confront in practicality, addressing the issues that contemporary health systems face. Regardless of the Moorean objection of the naturalistic fallacy, which in fact focused on ethical metaphysics and semantics, since we are here not debating the ethics of this motion, one would be hard-pressed to contend that all health systems would not at some point have to wrestle with the issues that two fundamental economic principles raise. These issues, namely that there is and always will be scarcity, and that hence we would have to optimize resource allocation and utilization, would invariably, result in the cross-interplay of factors, whose resultant ping even if so structurally benign, would be cacophonous. These issues explain at least in part, the observations made earlier regarding the ever-increasing health spending in many developed countries in particular, some with not much to show for it in terms of healthcare quality indicators. In other words, which underscores the point also made earlier about the heuristics value of characterized healthcare quality indicators, the chiasmic arroyo that we need to traverse needs to command more of our attention than it hitherto has. This is because it is our sojourn through it, which would involve complex, cross-domain negotiations, and exchanges, successfully or otherwise that would determine the influence that our interventions in the healthcare delivery enterprise, would have on the direction of its motion. It is okay to know the number of housing units that we would need for the homeless in our cities, as it is also infant mortality rates in our country, for examples. However, it is doubtful what impact this would have lacking the knowledge and appreciation of the underlying issues and processes behind infants deaths and homelessness, much more on how much we spend on health and welfare services. Yet, we not only want to provide these services, we want to do so efficiently and cost-effectively, as the two fundamental economic principles mentioned earlier dictate. However, we also want to do so, as we would discuss here later, also perhaps more fundamentally, due to derivations that our appreciation and acknowledgement of the core issues that the so-called 'is-ought' problem alluded to earlier regarding the naturalistic fallacy, would necessarily spawn. Again, we want to emphasize that our premise eschews any consideration of the goodness or otherwise of the motion referred to above as its driver, even if we concluded it is inevitable. Thus, on the other hand, at least from an ethico-moral perspective, we accept the fact that we predate language, hence value, even if the latter invariable colors, some would argue everything that follows, including scientific enquiry. This latter position is no doubt evident in the recent failure by some British scientists to receive the nod to produce a human/cow hybrid, which they considered would help in experiments that could lead to significant advances in the efforts to cure certain diseases. The direction of the 'flow' of scientific enquiry and knowledge is therefore clear, from this grounding of normative in positive arguments, as none on the ethical committee that ruled against the scientists probably had an iota of doubt regarding the potential of the hybrid regarding the expectations of the scientists. Thus, it is not necessarily of concern to us that whatever is unnatural is wrong, as with the example of the British scientists mentioned above or should it be, a clear reason why the issue of 'Appeal to nature' continues to plague us. One point here is whether or not, we need such an appeal, or if it was implicit in the unfolding evolution of our health systems, and even if indeed, what appeared to be implicit in fact is an artifact. Another is whether in fact, such considerations as above make any difference whatsoever to our efforts, which as we noted earlier would be evidently in between what 'is' and what 'ought to be' as far as our health systems go. Because of the blurring of this distinction as we noted with the case of the British scientists, where the 'philosophic' value of the evolution of scientific enquiry regarding the therapeutics for example, of those diseases, overruled whatever positive argument might be in their favor, we should focus on the transactions that enable us cross the 'chasm' successfully. This is okay except that it presents us with other dilemmas. One is that of determining the critical issues concerning the sustainability or otherwise of our health system in relation to that of our economic productivity and growth, which is evident from the patterns of the figures mentioned above, even if only from the perspective of the two key economic principles. The other, regarding the financing of our health systems, has to do with these principles too, albeit from a slightly different perspective, both however, ultimately convergent, predicated on again, core values, themselves, derivations from positive principles, the dialectics of both emergent in a continuum of multi-domain exchanges, whose very dynamics, constitutes the subject of this dilemma.

Debates over issues such as whether we should have only catastrophic health insurance, or whether we should have universal health insurance, not only indicate the need to address the roots of these issues, but by extension, the difficulty in resolving them, which more attention to the former would eventually achieve. If we concurred that we could not afford to continue to spend increasing portions of our country's wealth on health services provision, not to mention an investment on which we seem not to be getting much from in return, we have moved past any contention over the sustainability or otherwise of these health systems. We have also concurred by default the status quo, that our health systems are not efficient and cost-effective, not to mention not qualitative. Therefore, we have established the 'is', the way our health system is. What might, at first appear normative, regarding what it 'ought to be', essentially, is as we here hold, where it heads, regardless of us. This is the 'naturalness' implied earlier on, that to which we need not appeal. Regarding this 'is', the country notwithstanding, therefore, is the question of the acceleration or otherwise of this motorized entity, and its direction, forward, backward, or wobbly on a spot, which the nature and extent of our actions vis-à-vis the exchanges that characterize the healthcare delivery enterprise in effect dictate. Put differently, the longer we tarry over determining and executing the appropriate actions regarding those exchanges the likelier the motion would decelerate or wobble, which the longer it lasts, the worse it becomes, with the potential of the health system to cascade along a moribund path, potentially taking the economy in part, more or less with it. Why the 'normative' appearance is indeed, the 'is' predicates on the fact that it is irrelevant to our spending a given percentage on our health system whether, or not it is a good thing. Similarly, that such amounts could result in the cascade mentioned above, or hurt our ability to provide other essential services, and indeed, our economy, could be anything but whimsical. Yet, that we could modify the direction of the motion, underscores the blurring of the 'is' and the 'ought to be' mentioned earlier, the direction in which we modified it, essentially a product of the dialectics between the two, and this is the crux of the matter regarding the resolution of the dilemma also mentioned earlier. It underscores the need to dig deeper literally into the roots of these issues to resolve them, and pave the way for the motion of our health systems in the direction of acceleration forward, toward advancement, not regression, toward life, not death. The 'is'/'ought-to' interplay essentially starts as we first become beings, and then acquire values and culture. Even psychophysics tells us in receiver operating characteristics (ROC) that even we could err, differentiating weak signals, our conclusions regarding scientific observations, hence questionable, as the hullabaloo over the Fleischmann-Pons cold fusion experiment in March 1989, clearly showed. The question over what is fact or value could therefore, become quite moot. Thus, it matters little if the likelier tendency for an individual and by extension, the community, to seek the right to life rather than to death, is a fact, or something normative, since one could ground the premise of such a decision in what might look like either. However, that we are still here, as humans, and have been for a very long time, able to outsmart co-inhabitants of our planet several times our size and with strength that is far more superior, suggests the preference of our species for life over death, collectively. This very preference would inevitably drive the motion of our health services in the direction that it 'ought-to' go, which then in this instance is better still the 'is.' Since this 'is' applies to all human beings, barring any unforeseen natural catastrophe, it makes intuitive sense for any health jurisdiction, to establish immediately, the wherewithal to accelerate the motion in this direction of survival, not demise. The mechanics of this takes us into the realm of the political underpinnings of the roots of our assertion, of the inevitable motion of health systems in the direction of life, where again, we would encounter the critical issues involved in differentiating an appeal to nature from all else. As redundant as this distinction is as we have thus far seen, the need to acknowledge it requires an inclusive appreciation of its implications in relevant realms crucial to its applications in the variety of exchanges that pervade and determine healthcare delivery, and our interventions aimed at improving its quality, and moving our health systems in the direction of survival. Thus, each health jurisdiction would need to identify the issues that are important to the achievement of the dual healthcare delivery objectives (DHDO) of providing qualitative health services, cost-effectively and efficiently. These goals constitute the final common pathways in our efforts to move our health systems forward, as they address on the one hand, the issue of sustainability of the health system, and on the other, that of it financing, both one tier of the dual objectives. They also, in the other tier, address the issue of improving the quality of service provision. In determining these issues, health jurisdictions would realize the complex interactions of factors, health and non-health, which they need to deal with, some cross-territory, even international. The ability to achieve the DHDO would depend on how well the health jurisdiction tackles the challenges it would face in addressing the issues. The key issue in our moving the health system forward therefore is ensuring that we conduct this exercise as thoroughly as possible, a starting point that would determine the success of the other steps, and of our interventions, and one which needs to put the healthcare consumer at the center of the healthcare delivery scheme. This central place of the healthcare consumer has significant implications for our ability to achieve the DHDO. Yet the slow pace by healthcare professionals in many developed countries, of the adoption and utilization of healthcare information and communication technologies (healthcare ICT), technologies research evidence indicates could facilitate the achievement of these objectives, is instructive[6]. Given that we aim to improve the quality of services delivered to the healthcare consumer, the question of healthcare professionals embracing these technologies, is indeed, crucial, and underscores the need for health jurisdictions to understand the underlying issues and processes that hinder the achievement of the DHDO in their respective jurisdictions. However, many of these issues would have as earlier noted, national, and international flavors. Health jurisdictions would therefore, need to deal with them all, in whatever order they deem fit, all agents responsive in this regard, each addressing relevant issues within an established framework for example, whose basis also should be cross-sectional, rather than hierarchical. This presumes that agents would work within multilevel frameworks, these frameworks, becoming fewer, and more generic the higher the level. This would give agents at different levels the leeway to address problems relevant to them in improving healthcare delivery based on their intimate understanding of these problems, yet, would ensure that they work within a high-level democratic framework. It would be counter-productive, therefore, for such agents to operate a hierarchical control in their domains, in contradiction to this democratic framework, to which not just the health jurisdiction that is their principal, but the entire country in fact subscribe. This arrangement is crucial, and in fact, inevitable as evident in our discussion thus far. It is the organic driver of the motion referred to above, which moves not just the health system, but also all systems within a polity forward, backward, or around wobbling on a spot. It is thus the case that the increasingly perfect the process is, the faster it progresses, which makes the acquiescence to the democratic process strategic for not just health jurisdictions, but the entire country. It is in the exercise of the new knowledge that the healthcare consumer acquires for example as we rectify information asymmetry, that we could expect to hear his or her voice, key in exercising choice, itself key in assuring accountability, which helps to keep us all on our toes, literally, hence to move the system forward. This voice in addition would make valuable suggestions on improving healthcare delivery, and contribute to identifying the issues and processes that need attention, among others. This would make it more efficient and cost-effective to solve the problems that confront our health systems. Taking the residents of a particular health jurisdiction along for example in the efforts of the agents to tackle the jurisdiction's 'wait times' issues, could significant ease the problem in that jurisdiction. Understanding the efforts that the jurisdiction is making to recruit more family doctors, for example, could help the residents appreciate even more, the need to cancel doctor's appointments that they would likely miss, well ahead of time, so that the doctor could fill their place with someone else, which might significantly reduce 'wait times' in that jurisdiction. This again underlines the need for efficient and effective communication, among all healthcare providers. It might for example, also be possible to reduce 'wait times' in another health jurisdiction, with residents able to receive treatment on an ambulatory and domiciliary basis, with the necessary information networks in place to which not just doctors and other healthcare professionals, but also the healthcare consumer could connect. The question to what extent we should go in implementing these technologies is redundant if we considered the benefits derivable from so doing in the near and long terms.

Canada for example is investing billions of dollars via Canada Health Infoway to establish the architectural foundation for these networks, but would these massive investments not risk yielding limited benefits parts of the information communication circuit remains open? Why would we only want to benefit partially when we could in full, with all healthcare stakeholders hooked up to these networks? That the availability of current, and accurate patient information in real time to the doctor or other healthcare professional at the point of care (POC) could save many lives, and ensure the delivery of better services is not in doubt. Therefore, what we really should do is to ensure that this is the case, were we to benefit maximally from these technologies. This is a key issue to which the recent release by ten U.S. physician associations including the American College of Physicians and the American College of Surgeons, of eleven principles aimed at guiding health reform in the U.S., one of which is the availability of enough funds to support a 'comprehensive health information technology infrastructure and implementation, attests[7]. It is thus the case that our position might some would say conform to the classical consequentialist's, as opposed to that of a deontologist of similar mould. However, that we are in fact engaged in the moral validity of the motion described above, as opposed to its movement in any particular direction being a Kantian categorical imperative, is in fact also debatable. In the first place and as previously noted, the motion is not predicated on its goodness or otherwise, although the perception of some of its agents might be so. On the other hand, neither is it predicated on normative criteria. It is simply a motion that is part of an inevitable evolutionary process. Because its direction is not predetermined, to the extent that it could be in any of the three mentioned earlier, although even the seemingly static wobbly motion would eventually burn out, which given that of the backward motion, culminating in the same fate, vis-à-vis forward, potentially perpetual motion, the issue of predetermination again, is arguable. Viewed in this sense, one could argue that the inevitability implies determined. However, this again, is not the key issue, which is that, in general, we prefer to live than to die, even if as individuals, we must die, perhaps until we find the secret of longevity, and with life expectancy increasing, it seems at least that we have the potential to live even much longer than we currently do. This again, underscores the point that in the main life is preferable to death. Even despots must share the same preference, as evident in behaviors on their part that suggest that they must consider the perpetuity of their regime as given. The inevitability of the motion represents this preference played out in real life processes, and would play out, no matter the pace, even in despotic regimes. Thus, rather than agonize on ingrained intellectualism, we should disinvest the motion of attributes upon which it is inherently not dependent. It is just that for example no government that sits back as its domain crumbles would likely outlive that domain, even though both might perish, in the unlikely situation that this happens, although aided by external forces, such as natural and/or manmade catastrophes, it is quite possible. The example of Quebec, where a recent Statistics Canada survey, showed decreasing 'wait times', hence improving access to care, is illustrative[8]. According to the survey, published in mid-2006, across Canada, except Quebec, 20% of patients attempting to see a specialist in 2005, had some difficulty so doing, one in eight, in receiving non-emergency surgery, a similar number, less than satisfied regarding having a diagnostic test, and over 70% complained of excessive 'wait times.' In Quebec however, the median wait time for non-emergency surgery decreased by 50%, from 8.6 weeks in 2003 to only 4.3 weeks in 2005. The figures for other provinces remained unchanged, except for B.C., where median 'wait times' actually increased, from 4.3 weeks to 5 weeks, and Newfoundland and Labrador, form 4 weeks to 4.3 weeks, during the same period. The median wait time to see specialists in Quebec for a new condition was 3 weeks in 2005, same as from 2003, 4 weeks or more in all other provinces, actually increasing westward from Manitoba. Some query the objectivity of such telephone surveys, as in this telephone poll of 33,539 Canadians but it is difficult to ignore them in entirety. Do the reorganization of health services with for example in Montreal in late 2003, the coalescence of fifty-four health institutions into 12 regional health and social service centers, with the centralization, for example of cataract surgeries in three centers, with resultant goal to perform 20,000 surgeries annually exceed, surgeries performed actually 28,000, have to do with it? Does this not speak to the points we have made here about the evolution of the healthcare delivery motion being a function of the need for efficiency and cost-effectiveness simultaneously not compromising, but actually improving healthcare services, the achievement of the DHDO? Does that the province also optimized health spending since 2002, reallocating $47 million yearly for hip and knee replacements, and cataract surgeries, and devoting $50 million to reducing wait times for day surgery and those that warrant hospital stays, also not testimony to the inevitable operations of the two fundamental economic principles also mentioned earlier? Coupled with improved allocation and utilization of human resources, and of addressing such issues as appointments cancellation mentioned above, and list decongestion for a variety of reasons, for example, to address concomitant medical problems, including losing weight or reducing/quitting smoking, prior to certain types of surgeries, among others, these measures could also help other health jurisdictions reduce 'wait times.' Thus, health systems are in constant motion as healthcare delivery continues apace, what count regarding the outcomes of this service provision include, the quality, efficiency, and cost-effectiveness of the services delivered. It is regarding these factors we must concern ourselves primarily, the impetus for accelerating which crucially emerging from fundamentals we cannot ignore as they would reveal in-depth, the underlying issues that necessitate the attention to our health systems that they prescribe. Thus, debates in political circles regarding the establishment of specific policies at different levels to initiate and facilitate the promotion of the widespread implementation of healthcare information and communication technologies in the country seem convoluted bringing into the picture these fundamentals, whereas also easier to decide on the appropriate policies. How much government should engage in this exercise for example, could be crucial to the success of the initiatives, or otherwise. The lack thereof of government involvement on the one hand could result in the freer operations of market forces crucial to the achievement of the forward motion of healthcare delivery in the country is an assertion that could trigger intense political brouhaha. Indeed, as with other domains of our endeavor, the role of government in our affairs has been to say the least contentious, yet, needs resolution, starting with revisiting our conceptualization of the nature of the problem in the first place, which currently is essentially dichotomous. Do we for example have to see government's intervention as opposed to its graded, or non-intervention as incompatible, when in fact, nothing suggests they are other than the accumulation of conceptual misdirection that we have allowed to flourish? We have allowed this flaw to propagate itself by default, albeit this is not an excuse for contrition, but action. Given our preference for life rather than death, the onus is on us to perpetuate life that the other person also wants to, which makes it mutually beneficial for both to assure the survival of each other. The need for an external entity to secure this alliance is doubtful at this basic level, in particular if both persons had to contend with hostile creatures competing for limited means of subsistence. However, at a more complex level, and given the differentials in our intellectual endowments and personalities, matters could become very untidy, with again, collaborative efforts resulting in institutions that could ensure the survival of the alliance despite the gluttonous tendencies of some of the alliance's members, for example, could resolve. Since either member of the basic alliance could terminate the other, because of the perception of the terminated attempting to prevent the terminator from surviving, the terminator must consider it his or her right to survive. The need for such extreme or any action did not have to arise in this instance were the parties involved faithful to the agreement. Yet, that it could suggest that underlying the concept of right is its enforcement. In other words, that there is no right without enforcement capability, albeit potentially silent, or unenforceable because of weakness, as would be the case for the terminated in this example. Thus, it is clear that because of our preference for life, would be that for assuring it some way or another, more so in our much more, and increasingly complex world. The assumption, even for the basic dyadic is that the enforcing agency serves the purpose of the principals, the individual parties to the alliance, were the alliance to indeed, survive, let alone thrive. It is, we must also assume, that the existence of the agency implies the annulment of arbitrary termination by any or many agents by commission or omission due to a gluttonous tendency over weaker agents. This puts our conceptualization of the motion in direct collision with the classic tenets of utilitarianism, or even its broader conceptualization in consequentialism, which as John Rawls (1921-2002) eloquently noted in his *Theory of Justice* (1971), compromises fundamental democratic values. This was sufficiently important to warrant him stipulating, to ensure an unbiased agreement, or what he termed, 'justice as fairness', a 'veil of ignorance' on the parties in the alliance.

Rawls' 'justice as fairness', which predicates on the supremacy of each principal's right to crucial fundamental liberties for example, of thought and association being correspondingly available to another, and on equality of access to social and economic authority positions, inequality to be to the greatest benefit of the most underprivileged, underscores the integral ties between these fundamental issues. Thus, Rawls adduced moral backing for the sharing of each other's fate by principals being at the core of fair justice, and not equality in social status. This suggests that the task of the agency therefore is to ensure this happens, to prevent principals mauling one another in a 'state of nature,' the veneer of the present again, seemingly concealing what some would term, an appeal to nature, as in the 'social contract' to which Rawls' philosophy essentially owes its intellectual roots. Rawls' 'original position' implies acquiescence to rules, 'blind' to confounding factors that principals might have, for example, a particular advantage or setback, regarding a particular alliance or rule. His modification of the justice principle, emphasizing 'claim' by each principal, to a fully adequate scheme of basic rights and liberties, did not prevent his critics alluding to his ideas, a semblance to another comprehensive theory, even of the utilitarianism ilk, a doctrinal exercise in moral theorizing, not an exercise in autonomous political thought. Besides these criticisms, the idiosyncrasies in the latter formulation of Rawlian philosophy, in for examples *The Law of Peoples*, in which he postulated how 'well-ordered' peoples' society could be 'liberal' or 'decent hierarchical' underscores the need for the exercise, which engages us here, the perseveration of the 'appeal to nature,' in the evolution of the healthcare motion, crucial to address. This would elucidate the contemporary nature, extent, and potency of the Hobbesian Leviathan, in the healthcare delivery scheme, and indeed, in the interplay of this and other schemes crucial to the assurance and sustenance of the alliance, in its present form, and as it evolves down the road. We have concurred that the right of an individual to life is such only were it enforceable, and because it is, is a right, rather than just interest or desire. It is from this most basic of rights that every other right emerges. It also seems reasonable to assume that rather than being lawless monsters that cannibalize one another, we formed alliances that ensured our survival was why we have attained such distinction, intellectually and otherwise, an evolutionary process that would reverse itself were these alliances to break down, as for example, the terminator to keep terminating the weak, ad infinitum. Rawls' position on the justification of economic and social inequality therefore holds, and explains why as we have argued in this discussion, we need to consider the provision of qualitative healthcare to all as imperative, albeit a work in progress, an ideal to which we continually strive, one in fact attainable with us embracing the DHDO, for example. In other words, it is unlikely that the rich will continue to be richer and the poor poorer for ever, as this would be reversing the direction of the healthcare delivery motion mentioned earlier, in a recursive attrition, taking all of us along. Thus, it is not just the poor that would suffer the consequences of global warming for example, we all would, or that of the outbreak of avian flu in a remote Himalayan village, far from the metropolis in Europe or North America. It is therefore the case that there is no conflict between the principal and the agent, as neither has nowhere to hide when matters cascade down the path of death. Indeed, this would be the inspirer of the need for the establishment of the appropriate mechanisms and institutions to ensure the tendency of the breach of the principal-agent loyalty, with the interplay of stakes fostering potentially, multi-level loyalties, capable of compromising the alliances. Because our goal is to ensure the efficient and cost-effectiveness of the elements of the alliances, we would therefore in time have the mechanisms and institutions that could facilitate the achievement of these goals, one for example, ensuring that either principals or agents could exit questionable alliances and practices. Besides the need for information and knowledge to make these determinations in the first place being crucial, which highlights the points made earlier regarding the importance for us to rectify information asymmetry in the health and indeed, other sectors of our economy, the 'naturalness' of these processes is self-evident, which explains why we deem them inevitable. Thus, we could only prevent the reversal of the motion in a democratic milieu, where each person has a voice and could exercise his or her right to express his or her thoughts and associate freely with whoever shares or indeed, do not share these thoughts. These processes mean that like the 'original position', or 'state of nature,' we could and would ensure our survival with minimal intervention by an agent, since we have common fundamental goals, principals and agents alike. It would therefore, be evident for example that professional bodies are best able to regulate the practice of healthcare professionals than government, although government might have custody of crucial registration and other information that would contribute to professional bodies performing this task effectively and efficiently, hence the need for collaboration than the reverse. This underlines the flaw in the dichotomous conceptualization of the government's participation or otherwise in the healthcare delivery process mentioned above. What the processes motorizing healthcare delivery suggest is the need and in fact the likelihood of the motion being propelled by increasingly efficient and cost-effective mechanisms. The public service would therefore, increasingly embrace the principles of 'New Public Management (NPM), for example, the need for us to have sustainable economic growth and development, much more appreciated as a product of our ability to ensure justice. This would mean government even on its own recognizing the need for devolving many of what it currently does, focusing more on policy formulation, and sundry activities, the private sector, increasingly involved in essentially all sectors of the economy. The stress Rawls placed on basic rights would then coalesce with our need to strengthen our economy and address the issues of the underprivileged, including their health and welfare, within the public-private sector dyadic, in ways that would ensure the survival and progress of all entities involved. In other words, there is no conflict in the dyadic, that collaboration could not resolve and in fact, that is necessary in the first place in the true meaning of the word, not as we construe it in our atavistic contractarian/classical liberalism dichotomous mindset. There is thus, no subordination of individual liberty to Rousseau's (1712-1778) 'general will,' but rather an aversion for anarchy that we all in the main share, and that necessitates the preference for collaboration even within the context of competition. It is important for us recognize the workings of these processes, as we would then be able to appreciate more profoundly the roots of the actions that we take, or need to take in earnest, rather than wait. This is because we would still have to take them, lest we reverse the direction of the motion or at the very least, wobble, on the spot, neither of which would augur well for the country in an increasingly competitive global milieu, the tendency also to collaborate at this level notwithstanding. The 'mutual coercion, mutually agreed upon' that Hardin[9], noted, operational, at not just societal, but also inter-jurisdictional levels, as individuals and by extension their communities act in ways that ensure the preservation of their right to life, in a mix that effectively resolves the competition/collaboration conundrum implicit in the act. The more efficient and cost-effect the operations of the act, are, the more likely the achievement of the stated objectives that result ultimately in the preservation of that right. This is why as we have argued in this discussion, we should aim for increasingly efficient and cost-effective operations in our health services provision, as we would in so doing benefit maximally from the effects of health on the economy, which although both are a symbiotic dyadic, is in general more profound than vice versa[10]. We therefore, have much to lose not focusing on our health services, and making them perform better in both elements of the DHDO. In other words, and as Rawls emphasized, we should not focus only on economic efficiency, as this would not help us achieve the DHDO, which as the name implies, has two elements. The experience of the aftermath of large-scale hospital closures and the cutting back of funding for medical education in recent times in our country is instructive, as are those of countries that spend substantial amounts on health, such as the U.S., with returns, in the opinion of many examining health indicators, among others, not commensurate. The significant slowing of U.S. health spending growth in 2005, the slowest since 1999, according to the Centers for Medicare and Medicaid Services annual report, published in the January/February 2007 issue of Health Affairs[11], is impressive. Due to the fall in spending growth on prescription medications, as spending growth on hospital/physician and clinical services was the same as in 2004, it is however, only from the economic efficiency perspective, as not many would be that impressed by the achievements of the country's health system regarding the second element of the DHDO. This is the more pertinent considering that health spending in the country in 2005 rose 6.9% to nearly US$2.0 trillion, roughly US$6,697 per person, and the country spent 16% of its gross domestic product (GDP) on health, more than the 15.9% it did the previous year.

Thus, we need to focus on both elements of the DHDO, were we to achieve

the benefits of the motion of the health system, not precipitate its demise. It is interesting that the U.K's Royal Society in a report published on December 008,

2007, noted the wisdom in not discountenancing everyday technologies for examples, mobile phones, and personal computers in favor of large computer projects, such as the National Programme for IT (NPfIT), in the efforts to improve the NHS[12]. The report, 'Digital healthcare: the impact of information and communication technologies (ICTs) on health and healthcare,' also noted the slowness of the UK in adopting even the simplest healthcare ICT, which by so doing now, would better prepare the country to tackle future challenges, for examples, population ageing population, and the shortage of healthcare professionals, such as doctors and nurses. Thus, we actually have technologies now that we could use to jump-start the promotion of the widespread use of healthcare ICT that would complete the health-information network circuit. According to Professor David May of the Department of Computer Science at the University of Bristol and a Royal Society working group member, 'We set out to explore how future technologies could be used to improve healthcare, however it soon became apparent that existing technologies were not being used to their full potential. A variety of inexpensive, existing technologies can be adapted for a healthcare environment, for example, home security systems could be easily enhanced to incorporate personal monitoring to detect falls in the elderly, or mobile phones could be modified to analyze blood sugar readings to monitor chronic conditions such as diabetes.'[12] There is no doubt about the fact that such optimization of existing is a crucial components of the efforts on which we must embark to improve health services delivery, and move its motion forward. This is no doubt inevitable, and as professor May further noted, 'Over 15 million people in the UK reportedly live with a long-term medical condition such as coronary heart disease or diabetes. This figure is set to increase and is likely to place the health service under increased pressure. The growing variety of low-cost personal healthcare devices which can be bought over the counter or internet, such as heart-rate monitors and infection screening kits, will allow more people to manage their own health despite a potentially shrinking healthcare workforce.' This is so because funds would also be increasingly in shorter supply, and not just in the U.K., but also in our country, Canada. This is particularly the case as competition for other important programs, such as education and social welfare, which along with health the economic Historian and Nobel Laureate, Robert Fogel in, *The Escape from Hunger and Premature Death, 1700-2100*, considered the 'Big Three' that would dominate the 21st-century economy in many developed countries. In the Royal Society report mentioned above, Professor Frances Mair, working group member and researcher at the Department of General Practice and Primary Care at the University of Glasgow, also noted 'Simple technologies can make a real difference. Hospitals for example, are already text-messaging patients to remind them of appointments which saves hours of doctors' time in missed appointments. Web-cam consultations' could also enable healthcare professionals to monitor patients which chronic conditions such as asthma in their own homes.' There is no doubt that these observations apply to us here in Canada, and that, again, as noted in the report, we need to work toward overcoming the skepticism, hence seeming opposition towards the applications of these technologies in healthcare delivery common among patients and healthcare providers alike. This would require us addressing the multifaceted technology, ethico-legal, training and change management, and other issues that might be hindering the widespread diffusion of these technologies among different healthcare stakeholder groups, including problems, inherent in the healthcare ICT industry itself, such as project delays, product unreliability, not to mention those related to new systems' implementation and integration with legacy systems. We also need to formulate the necessary policies regarding the promotion of the pervasive use of these technologies, which along with the point mentioned earlier regarding inherent healthcare ICT industry problems, underscores the need for inter-sectoral collaboration between the public and private sectors, in various aspects of these efforts. Thus, we need to encourage not just doctors and other healthcare providers to embrace healthcare information and communication technologies, healthcare consumers, and other healthcare stakeholders, for example, the insurance industry, need to do likewise, how best so to do, which each jurisdiction would have to decipher. The fact is that we could hardly derive maximum benefits from the technologies were a complete information sharing circuit lacking. As Dame June Clark, Royal Society working group member, and Professor of Community Nursing at the University of Swansea noted, 'There is always an initial outlay of both time and money to establish any new method of working. Integrating technology at all levels of the healthcare system has the potential to save money in the end, but the real benefit will be better use of professional and patient time. District nurses spend hours a day traveling to visit patients when a call on a mobile phone would do the same job in a fraction of the time. Technology should never be a replacement for personal contact, but used as a complementary practice it will ensure the best use of limited resources,' the loop needs to be complete. We cannot ignore the importance of human activity in healthcare delivery even in future, and must relate that to the importance of the humans that these human healthcare professionals interact. In other words, we must do so at the functional and fundament levels, taking into cognizance, the stakes humans at all levels of the healthcare delivery enterprise have in its effective and efficient operations, which would reveal the profoundness of Dame June Clark's statement quoted above. In facilitating better use of patients and doctors' time for example, these technologies make the experience of time more meaningful, as it creates the enabling environment for both to derive fulfillment from the way they have utilized their time. The intense pressure of contemporary living, both in domestic, work, and other terms, and the psychological distress, which could transition to depression, perhaps even suicide, vis-à-vis the importance of the happiness, in fostering positive mental health and overall well being, is instructive. This is more so considering the significance of happiness, and by extension, health, for the economy. Incidentally, according to the World

Health Organization's World Health Report on the global burden of disease, depression is the principal cause of medical disability for individuals globally age 15-44, and it is common worldwide, leading to significant economic costs. Therefore, we need to do what we could to reduce the prevalence of depression, of which better time management is an important aspect, among others, and we need to emphasize the importance of the interdependence among us all, and the stakes we all share in ensuring that our society, and indeed, our country continues along the path of progress. This emphasis needs to start at a very early age, which means that a key task in our efforts to improve individual health and that of our society and country is to educate our peoples, at different levels. We need to provide them with the appropriate materials that would not only ensure that we all appreciate the stakes, but also could take crucial decisions in their best interests, and those of our country. We have seen thus far, the complexity of the tasks we have in improving our health services, yet perhaps the most basic thing we need to do in this regard is educating our peoples. This underscores, as we have done in this discussion, the crucial role information plays in these issues, and by extension, that information technologies could play in not just health, but education, and in other ways by which we could empower our peoples with the required information we need to change attitudes to health and healthcare delivery among all stakeholders. There is no doubt that we would need to appeal to the core values that bind us all in ensuring the success of these tasks. These values once understood in their fundamental and varied dimensions, would be the real drivers of the mechanisms that propel not just our health systems forward, but also our society, and indeed, our country, the need to do which could not be more urgent in our increasingly complicated contemporary world.

References

1. Available at: http://www.oecd.org/health/healthdata Accessed on January 14, 2007

2. Gerard F. Anderson, Bianca K. Frogner, Roger A. Johns, and Uwe E. Reinhardt, "Health Care Spending and Use of Information Technology in OECD Countries", *Health Affairs*, Vol. 25, No. 3 (May/June 2006): 819-831

3. Available at: No. 23 -Health Care Quality Indicators Project Conceptual Framework Paper (March 2006) Accessed on January 14, 2007

4. Donabedian A: *An Introduction to Quality Assurance in Health Care*. Oxford: Oxford University Press; 2003.

5. Institute of Medicine: *Crossing the Quality Chasm: A New Health System for the 21st Century*. Washington DC: National Academy Press; 2001.

6. Available at: http://www.healthcareitnews.com/story.cms?id=5298 Accessed on January 14, 2007

7. Available at: http://www.healthcareitnews.com/story.cms?id=6165 Accessed on January 15, 2007

8. Available at: http://www.macleans.ca/topstories/health/article.jsp?content=20060807_131475_131475 Accessed on January 15, 2007

9. Hardin, Garrett. The Tragedy of the Commons, Science, 162(1968):1243-1248. Available at: http://dieoff.org/page95.htm Accessed on January 17, 2007

10. Layard, Richard (2005). *Happiness: Lessons from a New Science*. New York: Penguin.

11. Catlin, A., Cowan, C., Heffler, S., Benjamin Washington the National Health Expenditure Accounts Team, National Health Spending In 2005: The Slowdown Continues, *Health Affairs, 26, no. 1 (2007): 142-153*

12. Available at: http://www.royalsoc.ac.uk/news.asp?id=5690&printer=1 Accessed on January 18, 2007

13. Fogel, Robert. *The Escape from Hunger and Premature Death, 1700-2100,*

A New-Stone Age

What has tax to do with healthcare delivery? The simple answer is that it is at the core of health financing. However, the question raises others about the proper role of government in healthcare delivery. From these emerge considerations, beyond merely ownership vis-à-vis efficiency and cost-effectiveness, of subtler issues such as the influence on this role, of competition and control in the health services milieu. Additionally, they alert us to the potential prospects and challenges of both the markets and of government in healthcare provision, which underline the increasing debates in many developed countries, including the U.S., and Canada, on the most appropriate approaches to, and the intricacies of healthcare financing that would increasingly require our attention in the years ahead. That how we finance our health services plays a crucial role in their accessibility for example, is not in question, many not able to afford health insurance, or lack access to health services to a more or less extent, even in countries with publicly funded health systems. In his weekly radio address to Americans on January 20, 2007, in a preview to his forthcoming Union address on Tuesday, January 23, 2007, President George Bush noted that reforming the federal tax code is potentially promising in making private health insurance more affordable[1]. The President plans to propose a tax reform, treating health insurance similar to home ownership, with as the current tax code for home ownership, enabling the deduction of the interest on mortgage from the owner's taxes, to provide a similar inducement for purchasing health insurance. In addition, he also plans to support states' efforts to tackle the uninsured and healthcare accessibility issues, his overall goals, to make health insurance more affordable, and to empower the healthcare consumer in making discerning choices regarding healthcare issues, in effect, to enjoy improved healthcare and healthier lives. These are indeed, noble objectives, but questions abound regarding the President's plans. Perhaps tax deductions, for example, might help those in higher income brackets for example, and not those who earn very little, who are essentially do not take deductions being on the short, not the long form itemized deductions, the very people who also could not afford health insurance in the first place, and for who the plans seemingly chiefly aim. In this regard, would the health insurance industry be the main beneficiary of the plans, as some would argue, the pharmaceutical industry is for the Medicare Prescription Drug Program? Is this then an example of the failure of both government and the markets mentioned earlier, and what could we do to prevent such failures, which many would contend are the chief reasons for the problems health systems face, not only in the U.S., but worldwide? Some would even question the rationale for government involvement in healthcare delivery, and if indeed, it should, in what capacity, and to what extent, the question of capacity, in another sense, that of the currency and adequacy for the management skills employed in the public sector, also crucial, to the eventual success of whatever role government plays. With regard, the latter sense, that public-sector bureaucratic monstrosity breeds sometimes-overwhelming inefficiencies, which compromise the quality of service delivery, including healthcare, is legendary in many countries, even the developed ones. Is this another reason, or in spite of which, we should jettison government intervention in the health sector, considering for example the enormous transactional costs resulting from these inefficiencies? This question is pertinent considering that such costs, as North (1990) noted, make up significant proportions of the Gross National Product (GNP) in developed countries[2]. In the health sector, for example, healthcare professionals in general have limited management and technical planning skills[3], which, could increase transactional costs and compromise the service delivery. Thus, many would argue that government participation in healthcare delivery should predicate, at the very least, on having the capacity to serve best in the capacity in which it operates. Besides the lack of the relevant skills set, the role diffusion that could complicate the scarcity of healthcare professionals inherent in them operating in management capacities would be an indication for such delineation of government participation for example. Yet, the flaws attributable to government participation in healthcare delivery have roots that are more fundamental than even those of the perhaps even more deficient management skills, evident in many health systems, of the non-medical management staff presumably with adequate management and technical training are. It is reasonable therefore, to assume that many management staff, medical trained or otherwise have enough management skills, but may be not enough to overcome the institutional challenges they face. These systemic challenges might in fact themselves not have emanated from just the health system, but imposed from outside, the outcome of the complex interplay of forces that bear in no small measure on the processes crucial to the success of the healthcare delivery enterprise. This also explains for example, why tax deductions could be such an issue in efforts to improve access to healthcare delivery, considering the other important uses to which governments put tax revenues, meeting the requirements of which competing interests could potentially scale back available resources for health services delivery. The potential effects of competition on healthcare delivery, also a crucial factor in the failure or otherwise of the markets, which in light of the call by some for limited government intervention in healthcare delivery creates a blind, prompting questions, of the subtle nature regarding the intercalation of government and private sector forces in healthcare delivery producing more viable dyadic. The roots of this perspective could in fact be just as profound as its potential outcome, whose unfolding would likely increasingly make redundant a dichotomous intellectualizing of an assumed government-private sector arroyo. It is hardly debatable that the professional bodies best able to regulate the conduct of their members, with government intervention in such exercises limited to establishing the framework and empowerment required for its exercise. However, such bodies might lack some vital information required for successfully regulating the professionals that government has, including data and information from various government agencies, hence even in this circumstance, the need for collaboration between government and these professional bodies, and between them, and the private sector, from where invaluable information could also come. Such inter-sectoral collaboration would more-imminently define the elements of healthcare delivery in the future, a new foundation that would reveal the inadequacies of the conceptual frameworks of the contemporary zeitgeist as it forges the path of progress. It would also be the veritable wellspring of the answers to questions of the hegemony of the health/allied industry-government complexes some apprehensively proclaim the bane of healthcare delivery. It would reveal for example the likely inevitable motion of the interplay of the dyadic of various kinds that these complexes spawn, in the direction that even their most vociferous nemesis yearns. This presumes the options of movement in two other potential, effective negative directions whose chances of occurrence are minimal, based on the core principles of the fundamental roots mentioned earlier, whose origin themselves, rooted in our beings, one would be hard-pressed to ignore. Considering that health services provision is for us, we should be at its core, a central position that nonetheless places us in jeopardy, its essential elements, crucial to the necessary outflow of the issues and their mechanisms from it whose ongoing resolution and efficient execution constitute the ingredients for the positive forward motion mentioned earlier, disregarded. That it is counterintuitive for example the mechanisms that perpetrate issues that would, even if in the long term, negate the entrenched interests that seemingly masquerade as such, and perplex their critics, equally oblivious, perhaps, to this veneer, belies the potency of the real issues operational in the final analysis. Thus, the health insurance and pharmaceutical firms would have elements of the processes involved in healthcare delivery working their ways not to make them work other ways in an inevitable collage of interests whose pursuit individually nonetheless creates a collective motion in an iterative heuristics with which we are yet fully conversant. This is why, at least in part, the dissonance of interests apparently becloud us, and partly also why the need to intensify our efforts to appreciate in full the underlying roots of these issues in accelerating this motion, becomes urgent, the consequences of delay in so doing, too difficult some would argue, to even contemplate. As the turmoil in many health systems currently evident, and which could potentially worsen given this delay shows, the need for such urgent action is in fact, imperative. That there is recognition of this need is obvious, considering the recent increased focus on health systems of the kliegs in many countries. What is somewhat enigmatic is the appreciation of its roots, which accomplished could be the compelling accelerant that our health systems need to progress apace in the desired direction.

Thus, with the expectation of the healthcare consumer ever more sophisticated, not to mention that of the entire system 'scarily' unforgiving, the pressure on our health systems to deliver would escalate to proportions many would actually find inspiring even if reluctantly at first. This initial awe, which we should expect, would ease with time, as our other initiatives in response to these pressures, for example, education, and skills training bear fruit, literally. The operations required on our part would hinge, therefore, on education, in general, and among others, to rectify the pervasive information asymmetry in the health system rooted in an atavistic paternalism, whose evolution reassuringly would coalesce with the mainstream developments moving the health systems forward, again, inevitably. Without necessarily ballyhooing it, since as we noted earlier the direction of the motion of our health systems is in the main tripartite, forward, backward, or wobbling on the spot, which could result eventually in motion in either of the other two directions, we could construe this as optional rather than absolute determinism. Thus, as we are the principals and agents in the healthcare transactions, depending on which side of the aisle we operate from at a particular point in time, the point is therefore to ensure that we play our part efficiently and cost-effectively. This explains the potential for the complexities of healthcare delivery, for example in the motives and outcomes of the interplay of the various forces operating on the health system, which stymie it unresolved. This situation calls for clarity in our conceptualizations of these roles, which would help define the subtleties of the involvement in them by respective healthcare stakeholders. We would then not just be concerned about ownership but also performance, at the highest level, both as we noted earlier dependent in the main on each other for expression. It would be thus, easier to re-conceptualize ownership in functional rather than structural terms, with even in publicly funded health systems the healthcare consumer, for example, having not just a voice, but exit options, in ensuring accountability in health services delivery, at the very least. Such potential, applicable to other healthcare stakeholders including the industrial complexes mentioned earlier and any other, underscores the cryptic underlying processes whose motion nonetheless is incredibly time-sensitive, and to which we necessarily subscribe, in moving healthcare delivery in one direction or another. In the public health sector, embracing and adhering to these re-conceptualizations would ferret these cryptic processes resulting in the potential coalescence with those in the private sector. In other words, with the healthcare consumer at the core of the principles guiding the operations in both sectors, the paradigmatic shift in the manner that the public sector conducts its operations might not be seismic, but would, nonetheless be catalytic, stimulating the sort of efforts resulting in the sharpening of the competitive edge in the private sector. This would increasingly be so as the dissolution of the hierarchical scaffolding of the bureaucratic behemoth that hitherto held sway reveals the tumescent antithetical foundation emergent beneath. The motion resultant streamlining operations, resource acquisition, allocation and utilization, for example, sets the stage for the healthcare dynamics of the new age, the efficiency and cost-effectiveness of government operations, a critical makeover that would redefine the nature and extent of its involvement in health services provision. It would be evident for example, why a health jurisdiction in Alberta should outsource orthopedic surgical services for a border town of a few thousand individuals to a hospital across the border in neighboring Saskatchewan province, rather than have patients in this Alberta town travel an extra hundred kilometers to receive treatment after waiting for six months. The evolution of the relevant institutions that would make transparent, the activities of the health jurisdiction, including for example, the opportunity for the residents of both towns to participate in deliberations regarding health services provision in their towns in a democratic arrangement that nurtures ownership and confidence in the health systems would make it that evident. This evolution would also make it evident the need for merging, even discontinuing services that are not viable, or not contributory to qualitative healthcare service provision in a particular health jurisdiction as deemed by this democratic horizontal consultation process. In other words, service provision would predicate more on rational considerations based on extensive multilateral consultations rooted in evidence emergent from an ongoing and contextual, process cycle analysis, each health jurisdiction operating within broad-based frameworks, themselves operating in a multilevel symbiotic dyadic. This analysis, a decomposition/exposition exercise that would dissect and reveal the sub-issues and processes germane to healthcare delivery in the health jurisdiction in question, enabling the determination of the required measures to modify them, to improve healthcare delivery, would engender a continuous quality evaluation that would ensure the perpetual improvement of service delivery. The overall result would be the achievement of qualitative health service provision, cost-effectively and efficiently, in other words, the dual healthcare delivery objectives (DHDO,) the necessary ingredients for moving the health system forward, in the context of its relationship to, and role in the country's economic growth and sustainable development. This is the grand outcome of the operations of the various forces operational in the healthcare delivery enterprise, which necessitates jettisoning the dichotomous mindset regarding the roles of government and the private sector in healthcare delivery mentioned earlier. This is because not only would the public sector assume new roles based on the outcomes of the analyses mentioned earlier, the tendency to, operate in capacities that it has the resources to best serve the capacity in which it operates as stated above would be empirical rather than whimsical. This would lead along the way to management innovations in health jurisdictions aimed at optimizing this tendency, including not just outsourcing services and the other examples mentioned above, but also competing with one another. This might not be, at least initially, at the intensity with which they would compete with healthcare providers in the private sector, or with which those in the latter would, with one another. The point her is that the revelation by a combination of factors in our time, including and in particular the changes in the perception of our world that education brings with it, the process, ongoing over time in a somewhat subterranean manner is becoming increasingly manifest, and as is inherent in the fundamental elements it represents, is inevitable. Thus, even if its form is new to us as it should, the elements of its transition, necessarily dynamic rather than static, that its direction rests squarely in our hands, explains the notion of optional determinism mentioned earlier, and the newness of the succeeding age we could expect to encounter, and which we should anticipate. This anticipation would not only make the transitioning smoother, but would make the direction of motion more determinable, hence the achievement of the fundamental objectives of the motion, realizable and quicker too. The unfolding of this process makes the pragmatism some would argue underpin it somewhat debatable, at least from the perspective of the common usage of the term to mean expediency. This is more so as the transition arguably involves elements of 'value', which introduces normative arguments grounded, as it seems in positive ones, a position articulated by Thomas Kuhn in his 1962 publication of *The Structure of Scientific Revolutions*. Nonetheless, there is no gainsaying the sense in the predication of service provision on the centrality of the healthcare consumer. Because the healthcare consumer seeks to achieve his or her fundamental right to life, that 'value', not a priori in the sense of Kantian categorical imperative, but the result of the conferment on evidence-based decisions that the vicissitudes of the observational capacities of human senses spawn, the cumulative value of the institutional prerogative that backs the decisions becomes important. As Richard Rorty also noted in *Philosophy and the Mirror of Nature* (1979,) we have varied 'discourses' available to us from which to choose to achieve ends, none preeminent, in effect linking Kuhn's 'scientific relativism' to classical pragmatism. This view coincides with our assertion of the three potential directions of the motion of healthcare delivery, each main direction with potential subsidiaries, whose characteristics the linguistic underlay of its discourse essentially determine. The extension of this position that we also hold, is the preference of mainstream humanity for the forward direction, although we see, even in contemporary times, the tendency for movement in the other two, in full, or in some flavor, with varying momentum, and even in the forward motion with similar characteristics. Thus, even in some countries with significant resources, health systems seem to proceed slowly, or sporadically, the accelerated epigenetic motion one would expect because of which abundant resources, apparently inconsequential in moving the health system forward at the pace it should. A delay in progress of this nature could have costly repercussions in many regards for even such countries, not least disruptive to the semantic evolution in progress in contemporary discourses, and that operates in tandem with the scientific, to create the pragmatic underpinning of the choices that ultimately move the health system forward.

The knock-on effects of such a delay on the body polity could have potential adverse impact on healthcare financing and the resource optimization, which could severely compromise healthcare delivery, and in turn the economy. Also unlike the opposing views of truth being that contributing the most good over the longest period to the community or the individual, akin to the tradition of Peirce and James, respectively, for example, we hold that the former is the inevitable extension of the latter, both an inseparable symbiotic dyadic. The applicability of our initiatives to the healthcare consumer, regardless of who is thus the basis, for the effects that we anticipate of these initiatives in the short and long terms on not just the individual, but also the community. Thus, we ought to formulate policies with the assumption in mind, tax deductions for example, based on the benefits on the individual's health, the appropriate allowances made for example, for those that complete the short form, if in fact any at all, as well. This is only when we could expect to derive full cumulative benefits from this initiative that would help to move our health system forward as the U.S. President no doubt aims to do, in making the tax reform proposals mentioned above, for example. The longer the positive effects the tax deductions on the individual's ability to purchase health insurance, for example, the more the health benefits that would accrue, which truth in essence becomes that of the community, which benefits immensely from it. Thus, it becomes easier for example for representative healthcare consumers on established town committees discussing issues pertaining to their health jurisdiction, to agree for example, on the need for some measures to reduce the costs to the health jurisdiction of managing smoking-related diseases, such as chronic obstructive airways disease or emphysema. They might also find it easier to concur on the criteria doctors could use to remove from hospital wait lists individuals whose overweight/obesity poses major surgical risk, hence need to lose some weight before reinstatement on the list. Thus, actions taken by the community based on truth that pertains to an individual become crucial in resource allocation and utilization that could determine whether health services survive in a particular health jurisdiction serving many. These actions also in fact do not hurt the individual but rather work in moving forward the healthcare delivery motion for that individual, some form of cost-sharing potentially discouraging smoking for example, or weight loss preventing potential catastrophe in surgery, not to mention its other health benefits. Delays in moving the health system forward, therefore, would make these processes difficult to achieve, the disruption of the semantic evolution of the principles that determine the applicability of 'superassertible' truth predicates, upon which the individual could base judgment on health issues, these principles not platitudinous, we hold, but hinged empirically. As Crispin Wright, who coined the term superassertibility, contended in his 1992 book, *Truth and Objectivity*, the predicate would be assertible in a particular information state, and endures, modifications to the state regardless, the recent decision by the French government to accord the status of a cultural industry to video games, as are already movies and music, instructive here[4]. This means that video games as movies and music would be eligible for tax breaks and government largesse to preserve French cultural heritage. Noting Culture Minister, Renaud Donnedieu de Vabres, 'I believe that a video game is a true creative work based on a lot of artistic talent, involving script writers, designers, and directors[4]'. Observers noted that France was base to three of the top ten video games firms, but competitive forces have compelled some such firms to shift operations abroad in search of cheaper labor, and a mix of culture and reduced taxes might help reverse this growing trend, or may be it is it too late, as some argue. However, with the plan including increasing the cultural content of video games, so that young people could learn some history and culture of France, to which we would add some health issues, the country is certainly likely to derive immense benefits from the exercise. With some video games already in the market that teach schoolchildren the history of France under Napoleon while they play, adding a note or two on the benefits of healthy lifestyles, or of the dangers of smoking and drug use would also play a significant role in truths about health for example that these young people grow up with. This would doubtless help inform their attitudes to health, which would reflect on their communities, the symbiotic dyadic mentioned earlier between the individual and the community motorized in earnest from an early age toward the positive direction that healthcare should head. The need for such early education regarding health issues is evident in the dramatic increase in the prevalence of overweight/obesity among children and adolescent in recent times, in both developed and developing countries. One cannot overemphasize the potential due to this trend for the earlier onset of the chronic diseases such as type II diabetes and their sequelae that currently result in significant disease burden, in human and material terms, and would therefore worsen cumulatively given the persistence of this trend. Added to the expected increase in the prevalence in developed countries that population would occasion, the need for urgent attention to these issues is not in question. This would constitute part of our efforts to keep the healthcare delivery momentum up as we indeed, should, to ensure the survival of these children, and that they have healthier lives. Here again, we see the community's truth predicates based on principles rooted in those applicable to each child, and which the child would be aware of for example, via education, utilizing, as France is doing, media they frequently use, the benefits of the individual/community dyadic to both evident in the community's overall health also thereby improved. The motion of healthcare thus heads forward, in the appropriate direction that would influence positively other key aspects of our existence, including the economy. It is therefore important that we focus on whatever efforts could result in fostering knowledge including rectifying information asymmetry in health and other domains. The significance of education in our efforts to facilitate the healthcare delivery motion is indeed, major, hence the need also for our heightened interest in the technologies, specifically information and communication technologies, which could facilitate the achievement of our goals in educating and informing all segments of society on health and related issues. With the healthcare consumer at the center of the healthcare delivery enterprise is the need for this consumer to have information and current and accurate information, too. This requirement for information is only age-dependent as far as the individual could not imbibe it until a certain age. In other words, our success in achieving our goals regarding information and knowledge acquisition requires starting the initiatives to help us achieve these goals as early as possible in the lives of healthcare consumers. Not so doing will only add to the latency in the healthcare delivery motion that results in health systems either progressing only sporadically, or in fact simply wobbling on the spot as mentioned earlier. The forward progress could recommence but the time lost could be punishing in many ways, for examples in human suffering and economic adversities at different societal levels, and domains, with individuals, corporations, small and large, and governments and their planned activities and programs, among many others, all potentially adversely affected. This not only underscores the coalescence of Rousseau's general, corporate, and personal will, it also therefore, as noted earlier, regarding the public/private dichotomy indicates that this is not the issue, as much as what the functionalities inherent in either could add to the motion that the dyadic could impel, healthcare delivery. The need therefore is to ensure that this motion is forward and that it is at the appropriate pace. Thus, we would have all agreed on the point that the stakes are high for all of us, public or private-sector based regarding the direction of this motion, and which because we could influence, we therefore, would. The point of this discussion is the need for us to have this appreciation, which would remind us therefore, in all we do of the need to contribute our quota to the achievement of the stated objectives. This makes the isolation of competition from the general scheme of the direction of the motion of not just healthcare delivery, but by extension, that of us all in general precarious, at least to the exclusion of collaboration. Indeed, it is evident of our lack of appreciation of some of the issues involved in the new foundation each transitional phase brings to the overall scheme. These include the key issue of the original dyadic that evolved voluntarily, which by its very nature required no agent to enforce, and which even with the emergent communities increasingly complex, invoked the preference of humans in the main to life. The starting point to appreciating our stakes in moving healthcare delivery forward therefore, is that of appreciating this preference and its meaning for the right to life. This right therefore does not derive from enforceability, but from an evolutionary commonality of preference, which makes the motion described above inevitable. It is therefore the reason that the institutions that nurture this preference survive and those that do not become moribund. This underscores the need for us to appreciate our different multicultural roots, and institutions, and to work towards their collaboration in achieving this ultimate commonality of preference, which therefore requires no enforcement. In other words, even in contemporary society, these institutions play vital roles, as they have been able to survive because they have kept faith with this precarious task, and would continue to adapt, even in our new foundation, lest they expire by attrition. It also means that so that we do not through our own errors delay the motion, we should acknowledge the fact that the fastest approach to averting such a delay is in promoting widespread information and knowledge acquisition. Hence, those communities, and countries that fail so to do risk costly delays, and coupled with the pace of progress in other communities and countries, their ability to compete effectively on the global arena more compromised. We are thus describing an inevitable competition/collaboration dyadic, evident even within households, but which managed effectively and efficiently could result in progress in the entity involved, on the one hand, and the inevitability of its motion in any of the three directions mentioned earlier on the other. The tilt of the dyadic would of course increasingly be in the direction of competition with transition from the household to the neighborhood, to the town, to state or province, and to country, for examples, but there is still going to have to be collaboration at every level for the motion at this level to move forward. The corollary therefore that the motion would either be backward or would wobble is true were the tilt to be reversed at each level, or the dyadic to be of an inappropriate mix, respectively.

The point here is the need for us to start to re-conceptualize health services

provision in novel ways, and to reorient policy formulations as well, to predicate our approaches to healthcare delivery on a new foundation stone in keeping with the realities of a new age. We would be able to see the need for actions on issues hitherto considered trivial but on which it might turn out, progress in our health systems would predicate, and to stay actions on others on which we currently invest inordinate resources with little if any resultant benefits. It would become clear the varieties of prescriptions we could give our ailing health systems to revitalize them, emanating from different levels of a dynamic interplay of forces, the potential for dominance by any ineffectual based on the appreciation in full by all of the fundamental roots of the symbiotic operations of the individual dyadic. The relevant institutions, processes and mechanisms emergent at each transition stage would add to the mix of checks and balances that ensure intervention by government in these operations, which would be clearly unstrategic even to governments, the way whose operations in other more appropriate domains, would be strategic and indeed, contributory to moving the motion forward. The primacy of healthcare in the evolution of society is evident from our discussion here, as is the need for the appreciation of this fact by individuals, even from a very early age. Yet, as is evident all around us, all is not well with healthcare delivery around the globe, with countries, in developing countries investing too little resources on it to achieve meaningful results, those developed, although investing substantially on healthcare delivery, relatively hardly faring better. When British Columbia reduced the number of health authorities from fifty two to six, slashed non-essential services, and streamlined Ministry functions, among others in 2003, these 'belt-tightening' measures in a massive, C$12 billion a year industry as they were certainly unpalatable to many in the province. Considering the keen interest among equally many in this province, the tussle reform efforts generate is evident. Yet, we need ponder the implications for resource allocation and utilization the recent analysis by the Canadian Institute for Health Information (CIHI) indicating a 17% increase in the number of surgeries performed in Canadian hospitals in the publication 'Trends in Acute Inpatient Hospitalizations and day Surgery Visits in Canada, 1995-1996 to 2005-2006.' The report indicates the performance of more day surgeries, a 31% increase in a decade, and less inpatient ones, a 16.5% decrease during the same period. Significantly, the data, adjusted for aging and population growth, also showed that a decline in the total number of hospital days in acute care hospitals, a 13% fall from 23.3 million to 20.3 million, during the same period, although the average stay in acute care hospitals in the country remained 7.2 days. Do these figures indicate the trend towards more efficient service allocation and utilization, and if so, would continue to see evidence of such efficiency in other service areas, or not? If we were to reckon based on our assertion of the inevitability of the evolutionary path that our health systems would take, the answer would no doubt be affirmative. In fact, what we should aim to achieve is the quicker achievement of this efficiency in all aspects of healthcare delivery, indeed, overall, the achievement of the dual healthcare delivery objectives (DHDO), and we should seek the best and fastest approach to doing so. This means, and as we noted earlier, eschewing entrenched positions on health financing, and re-conceptualization our concepts of the elements of health services delivery, an exercise crucial to our ability to see and adopt the required approaches to realizing our goals. There is no doubt that health financing is one key element. With the re-conceptualizing of this element would be the revelation of novel ways to address the issue, including the co-habitation of public and private health financing. The point here is that what should be important to us is the achievement of the DHDO. In providing qualitative health services to all Canadians, simultaneously reducing health spending, we would not only be realizing the fundamental principles inherent in the Canada Health Act, we would be saving significant funds. We could use these funds for example, in improving education at all levels, and facilitating the achievement of the information and knowledge acquisition relevant to the understanding in full moving healthcare delivery, and indeed, Canada forward from an early age, and indeed, throughout the life cycle. This is besides the fact that with the health of Canadians at its peak would be the economy of the country too, a situation that would sire further improvements in both in a characteristic symbiotic dyadic of which sort, many of the factors operational in not just healthcare delivery, but also other aspects of our life are. We would be doing the country immense good therefore, refocusing on achieving the DHDO rather than on which of public or private health financing best suits the country, in particular if with neither the potential to not really deliver the health services that Canadians need, worse still even with increasing amounts of their resources infused into financing these services. Thus, we could allay the anxieties of the protagonists of public health system financing, including that, private health system in parallel with Medicare would make health services increasingly inaccessible to the poor, and those unable to afford private healthcare. The fundamental reason for this assertion is that a parallel private health system in Canada would deplete the public health system of already scarce work force, including doctors and nurses and other healthcare professionals, offered more pay. Even if this were the case, it would likely be a temporary setback, one in fact, the public health system could avert by embracing the same principles that enable the private sector afford the offers that might pull health professionals in their direction. In other words, the more competitive our public health systems become, the less the likelihood of the feared exodus into the private health sector. Vital to the public health system being more competitive is to acknowledge that the healthcare consumer is at the center of the healthcare delivery universe. This would ensure that policies and the initiatives emanating from them are consistent with ensuring that the healthcare consumer receives the best quality healthcare, and that avenues exist not just for the healthcare consumer to participate in and influence healthcare, but also to have options regarding care. Part of the effects of participation and choice would be to promote accountability and transparency in the healthcare delivery enterprise. Indeed, by adopting more rigorously key elements of New Public Management (NPM), whose key elements incidentally include transparency and accountability, public health jurisdictions would be more competitive, hence able to withstand competition within and outside the public health system. The increased efficiency that would result would permeate all sectors of healthcare delivery, the changes brought about reflecting in the significant reduction in transaction costs of healthcare delivery without compromising the quality of healthcare delivery, because the achievement of this qualitative service is implicit in the supremacy of efficiency in the operations of all is sectors. Thus, commitment to improved efficiency would lead to superior service quality, and decreased costs, or put differently, the achievement of the dual healthcare delivery objectives (DHDO.) To improve efficiency then, we need to equip the healthcare consumer with the relevant information and knowledge to assist in making discerning decisions capable of ensuring qualitative participation, and rational choices. It is also important for health sector-operatives at all levels, to have the current and relevant data and information that they need for enhanced productivity, including which information communication and sharing would spawn. Therefore, information and knowledge acquisition and appropriate utilization are major aspects of improving efficiency in health services provision. It follows that the more efficient the exercise, the more efficient the health system is, and a more efficient health system would likelier be more competitive. The point here is that competition is the key to survival in the private health sector. This means that in addition to competing with others in the private sector, healthcare providers in that sector would have to compete with an efficient and cost-effective public health system. This competition would effectively stem the 'exodus' mentioned above, as the private sector increasingly pays less to healthcare professionals due to the falling prices of healthcare delivery that market forces would inevitably compel. In both the public and private health sectors, information and knowledge acquisition and utilization are important for efficiency. In both sectors, it would be increasingly important to implement the appropriate technologies to rectify information asymmetry and to facilitate information flow. Additionally, it would be even more important for the public health sector to implement healthcare ICT to be able to compete with the private sector, which would, run as businesses typically are, would have little if any choice in implementing these technologies, to survive in what would be an intensely competitive environment, let alone thrive. They would need these technologies as elements of their value propositions to offer enhanced services that could differentiate them from their competitors, increasing patronage, hence profitability. The public health system is going to need to initiate competitive value propositions akin to those offered in the private health sector for it to retain patronage, hence remain viable, economically, and otherwise. This is going to result in public health systems, again as private health systems would 'naturally' do, choose which services to provide most efficiently and cost-effectively, and this is a key point, one that is at the core of our proposition here of the redundancy in dichotomizing health services delivery in our country. The need for public health systems to make these choices means devolution, in a manner of speaking by proxy, of certain services to the private health sector, which suggests the natural and inevitable evolution of this latter sector in our country's healthcare delivery landscape. Which and how many services particular health jurisdictions decide to keep or jettison would depend on local factors these jurisdictions consider crucial to their survival. This means that not only would this private health sector evolution vary in the nature, number and size of services 'devolved', it indeed, means that some jurisdictions would proceed with this devolution at a faster pace than others, but all, eventually would. These are important issues that we need to start to pay serious attention to from now and not, perhaps conveniently for political expediency choose to ignore, or delay acting upon for any other reason. As we noted earlier, such a delay could end up being costly to the country, in health and economic terms, and in our ability to compete effectively in an increasing global world stage.

These issues also show the importance of health in our affairs and the need for us to acknowledge this fact and address it as urgently and comprehensively as possible. In the first place, we must take the evolution of Medicare more seriously, and examine its potential, long-term to change in ways we can hardly imagine as constituted. This scrutiny would enable us prepare for these changes adequately, hence not be caught flat-footed, literally, when they eventually occur. What for example would be the effects of population aging on this evolutionary process, and would it accelerate or decelerate it? How would these effects play out in relation to health financing, and on our economy, with for example, services for the elderly shifting in one direction or the other between the public and private health sectors? Could certain initiatives, for example, more efforts focused on preventive care steer this direction, also one way, or the other between these two healthcare delivery sectors? These and other questions would be important to answer lest we confront challenges that could overwhelm our health systems, both private and public. If the former, in the sense of falling prices for services that could attract an increasing number of clients, with many and complicated health issues, and the latter, the potential for service over-utilization for which capacity might be lacking. It would be much more accurate to plan for resource optimization in both sectors examining in detail, the requirements for services that would be necessary based on projections of the magnitude and nature of our population aging. Each health jurisdiction in the country would have to conduct this exercise, which would reveal the services it should rather devolve, considering a variety of factors, including the size of the population served, the availability and types of healthcare professionals, its budget, and the availability and types of private health services, among others. This also underscores the need for and the inevitability of collaboration even in competition that we mentioned earlier, as in this instance, it would serve both sectors well to collaborate on service provision for the health jurisdiction in question. Furthermore, it underlines the significance of the central role the healthcare provider would increasingly play in health services delivery in our country. This is because such collaboration without the input of the healthcare consumer would likely come to naught. It certainly makes sense for any entity planning health services provision for a community to know the needs of that community, which is where the consultation based on democratic principles with the healthcare consumer is crucial. This again highlights the need for us to rectify information asymmetry and make it possible for the healthcare consumer to make meaningful contributions to such collaborative efforts. Such enlightened contributions would give the healthcare consumer a sense of ownership in the health affairs of his or her community. This ownership would in turn promote responsible and discerning service utilization, which would result not just in cost savings, but more efficient service delivery, for example, health consumers canceling well in advance doctors' appointments that they know they would likely miss, reducing the 'wait list'. By reducing the 'wait lists,' healthcare consumers would receive treatment more promptly, which would reduce morbidities, and indeed, mortalities, reducing the human and economic burden of infirmity. It is therefore clear that key attributes of a committed effort to anticipate the potential future challenges to our health systems, and to sustain their ongoing quality improvement measures are information and knowledge acquisition and utilization in either or both of generating over time an informed healthcare consumer populace, and in information communication and sharing among healthcare stakeholders. The former would be part of our general efforts at improving education in the country, the latter, of improving the availability of critical patient at the point of care (POC), for example, and in general enhancing communications and productivity within health systems and between them and other systems, external yet crucial to their survival. We should promote thus, as part of these efforts, the widespread diffusion of healthcare information and communication technologies, as they are the core of efficient and cost-effective mechanics of information husbandry and utilization in the most valuable ways to assist us in achieving the dual healthcare delivery objectives. The tripartite of education, health, and healthcare ICT, are going to be the key drivers of the evolution of our health services. We need to begin to pay closer attention to all three in a new age, that antedates another, which other itself the latter would in a continuous process, which as we noted all along, we could choose whose direction, and we should, driving forward the motion of all three, hence that of our economy, and of our country.

References

1. Available at: http://www.marketwatch.com/news/story/story.aspx?guid=%7B8F766666%2DB698%2D4B2F%2DA674%2D0515FE37A1F5%7D&dist=rss Accessed on January 20, 2007

2. North, D.C (1990) Institutions, Institutional Change, and Economic Performance. Cambridge University Press, Cambridge.

3. Mills, A (1997) Improving the efficiency of public sector health services in developing countries: bureaucratic versus market approaches. In Colclough, C. (ed.) Marketising Education and Health in Developing Countries. Claredon Press. London.

4. Available at: http://news.bbc.co.uk/go/pr/fr/-/2/hi/europe/6272301.stm Accessed on January 21, 2007

Conclusions

Healthcare in Canada is an integral part of our culture. We value our health in ways outsiders might not fully comprehend. It is important that we not only continue to cherish our health, but also to ensure that the services that we have established to help us keep our health in excellent form are qualitative and cost-effective. As we have seen in our discussion in this e-book, achieving these goals, require an in-depth appreciation of the issues involved, many non-health in nature, yet have profound effects on the direction in which our health services head. No doubt, our ability to couple this appreciation with apposite policy formulation and implementation at different levels of our health jurisdictions would facilitate the achievement of the noble healthcare delivery objectives that we set out accomplish.

That our health services would continue to evolve is inevitable, yet as we noted in our discussion here, maneuverable. This is a key point that we also need to appreciate, as it is clear thereof that the direction in which healthcare delivery in Canada evolves depends on our actions and even inactions. It is also important to know that even if we worked toward a positive direction, the pace at which we do so also matters, any delay in moving healthcare delivery forward fraught with the danger of compromising not just the overall health of our peoples but also that of our economy, and its competitive capabilities on the world stage. This makes it our responsibility to ensure that every Canadian receives as needed, qualitative health services, and further, that we do not spend disproportionate amounts of the country's wealth on health services provision in the process jeopardizing not just our ability to fund other essential services, but also our economic growth and development.

Healthcare provision is Canada would therefore have to be a balancing act in which the factors operate such that we achieve our stated healthcare delivery goals. We would have to make the necessary adjustments rather than wait for them to happen in their own time, as they would, which our discussion in this e-book clearly revealed. As earlier noted though, why should we even let this happen, when we could avert the potentially significant costs? In other words, a key aspect of our aim in this e-book is to emphasize the need for reorienting ourselves regarding our approaches to healthcare delivery, to recognize the inevitability of the motion that we have described and the futility in dichotomizing health services provision. Rather, we should reset our objectives to embrace achieving the dual healthcare delivery objectives (DHDO) primarily, and their sub-goals, secondarily, and to reflect our new mindset regarding the forces driving our health services and to what extent and how we could be at the driver's seat.

Copyright Bankix Systems Ltd January 26, 2007

www.ingramcontent.com/pod-product-compliance
Lightning Source LLC
Chambersburg PA
CBHW030624220526
45463CB00004B/1405